D0413175

Learning Journals

A handbook for reflective practice and professional development

Second edition

Journal-writing is an increasingly common technique in education, personal and professional development.

Fully updated with important new theory and practical material, this second edition of *Learning Journals* offers guidance on keeping and using journals and gives step-by-step advice on integrating journal-writing on taught courses, in training and professional development, and in supporting personal development planning (PDP) activities. Essentials covered include:

- the nature of learning journals and how we learn from them
- the broad range of uses of learning journals, including portfolios and personal and professional development
- the depth and quality of reflection in learning journals
- the assessment of learning journals and reflective writing
- the use of narrative and story-telling techniques in journals.

With useful exercises and activities that enhance learning journal work in a structured manner, *Learning Journals* is invaluable reading for teachers and students in higher education, for all professionals, particularly those working in the health services and business and training, and for all those who want to learn more about keeping a fulfilling personal journal.

Jennifer A. Moon researches learning at the Centre for Excellence in Media Practice, Bournemouth University, and is an Independent Consultant.

Learning Journals

A handbook for reflective practice
and professional development

Second edition

Jennifer A. Moon

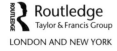

Routledge
Taylor & Francis Group

LONDON AND NEW YORK

This edition published 2006
by Routledge

First edition published 1999
by RoutledgeFalmer
2 Park Square, Milton Park, Abingdon, Oxon OX14 4RN

Simultaneously published in the USA and Canada
by Routledge
270 Madison Ave, New York, NY 10016

Reprinted 2007 (three times)

Routledge is an imprint of the Taylor & Francis Group, an informa business

© 1999, 2006 Jennifer A. Moon

Typeset in Times New Roman
by Keystroke, 28 High Street, Tettenhall, Wolverhampton
Printed and bound in Great Britain
by Cromwell Press, Trowbridge, Wiltshire

Apart from any fair dealing for the purposes of research or private study,
or criticism or review, as permitted under the Copyright, Designs and
Patents Act 1988, this publication may only be reproduced, stored or
transmitted, in any form or by any means, with the prior permission
in writing of the publishers, or in the case of reprographic reproduction
in accordance with the terms and licences issued by the CIA.

British Library Cataloguing in Publication Data
A catalogue record for this book is available from the British Library

Library of Congress Cataloging in Publication Data
A catalog record for this book has been requested

ISBN10: 0–415–40376–6 (hbk)
ISBN10: 0–415–40375–8 (pbk)
ISBN10: 0–203–96921–9 (ebk)

ISBN13: 978–0–415–40376–4 (hbk)
ISBN13: 978–0–415–40375–7 (pbk)
ISBN13: 978–0–203–96921–2 (ebk)

Contents

Preface

The content of this book is largely introduced in Chapter 1 along with a general introduction to the topic of learning journals. This preface represents a few notes on how this book might be read.

A book on learning journals might be looked at by those interested simply in the nature of a pedagogical tool that promotes learning. It might be read by those interested in the theory of how one learns from journal-writing or those who want to write a journal for themselves for personal or professional development reasons. It might also be read by tutors, who may have decided that tomorrow they will confront their class with the task of starting journals, and want to know what to do. From experience, there is a need for information about assessment of journals too.

There are many ways in which this book might be read, only one of which is the cover-to-cover mode. While the chapters are arranged in a logical sequence for the reader of the whole book, it is possible to glean more specific information by reading a selection of chapters of immediate relevance. The chapters are relatively self-contained, and, in particular, that applies to the more practical approaches of the last few chapters. The cost of self-containment is a little bit more repetition than there would otherwise be.

With reference to terminology, we have adopted the term 'learning journals' but there are many alternatives that involve the same activity (see Chapter 1). The book contains much information and many ideas that would support those working as tutors or learners with 'portfolios' – often the terms 'portfolio' and 'learning journal' overlap in use.

The book is well referenced: there are not many other substantial bibliographies on this topic and in this respect it represents a sourcebook. The broad range of references supports those using learning journals for personal use or for use with others. Many of the references provide examples of how journals have been employed in different contexts and therefore they complement the material contained herein.

In this second edition of the book, we have recognized that the use of journals has become much more widespread since 1998, when the first edition was written. At that time, the idea of a learning journal was relatively alien to most teachers in higher education and many of the examples were from the 1980s in the United States. Now there are relatively few subject areas in which there is not local documented use of learning journals of some sort. In addition, the advent of personal development planning/profiling (PDP) in the UK has meant an almost general acknowledgement of the value of reflective activities, if not journals as such. Many of the tools for personal development planning are, in effect, highly structured journals.

There are three new chapters or sections in this second edition. The first develops the consideration of the relationship between journals and the process of learning. The second pursues the idea of reflective learning by seeing it not just as something that happens or that does not happen, but as a capacity that has superficiality (when it is descriptive) or depth. This new thinking provides a more rigorous manner in which we can view learning journals. The same thinking has led to a form of exercise to help learners to start their reflective writing and to 'deepen' it, thereby improving its quality and – we assume – the quality of learning that can result. Some of the work on reflective learning is based on a book by the author that is devoted to the exploration of reflective and experiential learning (Moon, 2004a).

The other new chapter is on journals and their relationship to story and narrative. This has been written in order to recognize the significance and relevance of the currently growing literature on narrative in professional development, in business settings, in sport and education for journal-writing – as Rainer puts it, to recapture some of the psychological nurturing that can result and which has been gained from myth and ritual in the past (Rainer, 1978). Much journal-writing is, in effect, the writing of personal story.

The third new section consists of resources that can be used to aid the development of reflective writing. It consists of photocopiable exercises and related support material. In addition, this new edition also addresses an important topic on the ethics of the use of learning journals in education (within Chapter 9).

The book has largely been rewritten. It also contains more practical activities and materials that can be used directly with learners or by learners who use a journal (Chapter 13).

Chapter 1

Backgrounds

An introduction to learning journals

Introduction

We start by looking at the term 'learning journal' and the boundaries of the definition that are adopted for this book. We ask 'why write a journal?' and use some comments from those who write journals or who manage journal-writing in educational situations to illustrate a range of enlightening and creative aspects of the process. The next section roots the discussion in its past and present contexts. We sketch in the manner in which present ideas of learning journals have been developed and how journals become a topic in their own right in academic and educational literature. There is, too, a personal context for the writer's chosen subject matter and for this book. It describes how the book came to be written and how it relates to a more than an academic interest in the human process of reflection. With some roots to the topic of learning journals in place, we can begin to widen the discussion in the last section, towards an anticipation of the rest of the book.

What is a learning journal?

A learning journal is essentially a vehicle for reflection. Probably all adults reflect, some more than others, and for those who do reflect, being reflective can represent a deeply seated orientation to their lives. For others, the process would seem to come about only when the conditions in their environment are conducive to reflecting, perhaps when there is an incentive to reflect, or some guidance or a particular accentuation of the conditions. A learning journal represents an accentuation of those right conditions – some guidance, some encouragement, helpful questions or exercises and the expectation that journal-writing can have a worthwhile consequence, whether during or at the end of the process, or as a result of both.

There are many different words that are used to describe what we are calling 'learning journals'. They may be called 'diaries', but not the sort of diary or calendar that notes dates for events (that is, the kind that is carried in a handbag), though they might do this as well. They may be called 'logs' or 'learning logs', but they are not logs only in the sense of recording data at particular points in time or place. An example of the latter would be a ship's log in which data is written at fixed points in a ship's passage. A learning journal is very likely to include some factual recording about place or time but for the sense here, it means more than that. Sometimes a learning journal, as we have said, is the same as a personal development plan, a 'progress file' or a record of achievement (NCIHE, 1997; Cottrell, 2003). It may, likewise, coincide with many aspects of a portfolio in which a range of learner's work or evidence of work is accompanied by a reflective commentary. There are other words that have been or may be used to describe broadly the same activity as the keeping of a learning journal. Old terms are 'commonplace' or 'common-day' book (Rainer, 1978) which could be descriptive or might have a more constructive purpose. 'Think place' or 'think book', 'notebook' and 'workbook' are other terms that arise in the literature. There are some other words such as 'ponder' that might be engaged here.

Precisely defining words – such as 'journal' – is unhelpful here because it is a situation in which the creative development of personal terms is an aspect of the very process of reflective learning. In this book, by 'learning journal', we refer to an accumulation of material that is mainly based on the writer's processes of reflection. The accumulation is made over a period of time, not 'in one go'. The notion of 'learning' implies that there is an overall intention by the writer (or those who have set the task) that learning should be enhanced. For this reason, the descriptive diary that never goes further than describing events is not part of the subject matter of this book. Within this generalized form that we describe here there are vast creative possibilities with many illustrations of these in this book.

So we are not talking about something with a fixed definition here. The definition has fuzzy edges. For example, the idea of writing a journal mostly implies an activity that is personal and relatively solitary, but one form of journal-writing involves two or more people who construct the same document. 'Dialogue journals' represent a written conversation between two or more people, each responding to the other's entries, usually around an agreed topic, though, as in the nature of any conversation, the topic may shift and a new one may be introduced. Shifting on in meaning a little brings us to email conversations, and the various software mechanisms whereby a large number of people can read or contribute to a discussion, with the topics organized into strands (e.g. blogs and wikis).

Another example of activity that may or may not fit our notion of 'learning journal' is the autobiography. In the past few years the literature on story and narrative in education and professional development has increased greatly (e.g. McDrury and Alterio, 2003). As an example, many teacher education programmes utilize autobiography as a means of exploring students' pre-course conceptions of teaching, teachers, school and other concepts that may distort their new role as teachers. Sometimes this form of work would not be sufficiently continuous in time to fit our definition, or it may be an exercise within a learning journal.

An aspect of the definition on which we have not yet expanded is the form of expression of the reflection. It is easiest to think of journal work as written and often it is handwritten. A pen and notebook may not now be vastly more convenient to carry than a palm-top computer, but they are still cheaper, and for many people there is something more expressive about a favourite pen than a keyboard. Electronic journals have advantages, and one, in particular, is where parts of the journal can be communicated to others by email – such as in the case of a dialogue journal or the discussion lists that we have mentioned above.

Verbal reflection can be recorded on tape. Audio-diaries have become relatively common on radio. Here they might take the form of the individual making regular recordings during a journey – or during the experiencing of an event. As this is written, an audio-diary broadcasted in the summer of 2005 on the BBC comes to mind (BBC Radio 4, 8 August 2005). It was made by a relatively unknown Scottish band, the members of which were suddenly drawn into 'top of the charts' status in Serbia. They reflected on their journey to Serbia across Europe in an old van, the brief experience of stardom and the trundle back into everyday life.

We do not assume, either, that journals are always verbal. Words can be mixed with drawing or drawing may predominate. Learning journals are close or coincide with the idea of the artist's notebook. In architecture or art, the noting and exploration of graphic form over a period of time might be the subject of a journal and parallel ideas might be applied in music and it may even occur in dance and acting. These different forms of recording in a learning journal need to be borne in mind when reading this book but, for convenience, most of the text will refer to the written form of recording.

The subject matter of journals – what it is that people are writing and thinking about in their journals – will be covered in many areas of this book. For convenience we divide the main approach to the subject matter of journals into three areas – personal development, journals in formal non-vocational education and in the context of professional education and development. There are large areas of overlap of likely subject matter in these areas. For example, few would separate personal development entirely from professional development (Harvey and Knight, 1996). Equally, professional or vocational issues may well emerge in a personal journal but are also sometimes of relevance to a student's development within his or her discipline.

Beyond the three big categories here, however, there are some surprises in the literature. While it is clear to see that there is no limit to the day-to-day subject matter of a personal development journal, there also seems to be little limit to the subject matter about which journals may be written in the field of formal education. This book will discuss the use of journals in over 30 disciplines in formal education. These disciplines range far from the humanities and arts, where the home of journal-writing might seem to be, to the sciences and applied sciences of engineering and computer studies. It is useful that basic subject matter inspires the development of different structures for reflection and writing and these different structures can then be adapted and applied elsewhere. Many of the exercises that are described in the last two chapters of this book have been adapted from specific applications in other contexts.

Another major variable in journals is their structure. A simple personal learning journal may be no more than a recording of the features of the day with reflective commentary and consideration of the issues raised. However, an extreme example of a structured journal is also one most often focused on personal development. Progoff's 'Intensive Journal' (see p. 132) consists of 19 sections, many of which have associated methods recommended for their entries (Progoff, 1975). Between these extremes, there is wide variation, which is often defined by the subject matter or the purposes of the journal. For example, in formal education, journal entries may often relate to coursework – the content of lectures and reading work or entries may be required to follow a sequence of questions that are designed to structure reflection. Often, however, students who are guided in some of their entries are encouraged also to write freely in another section. As we noted, we have personal development planning that links the academic experiences of a student with her broader experiences of being a student and with her developing aspirations for career.

The question of audience for the writing of a journal raises some interesting issues. It has three aspects that may be linked. First, for whom is the journal being written, in the sense of who is it who has decided that it will be written? (Is there any choice not to write it?) Second, who will see it – will it be assessed and seen by another in that context or will it be seen by a tutor who will ask only helpful questions to guide reflection to unconsidered issues? Will it be seen by peers? Individuals may choose to share aspects of their journal with another for mutual benefit or for their own benefit. There are benefits from sharing journal-writing, but it can be risky, too, and the knowledge that one is sharing can distort the process of writing. The third aspect, of audience, may remain in a conscious or unconscious state with the writer. Writers of personal journals may become aware that they are writing for a particular audience – perhaps their children, or others who may see the journals after the writer has died. Thoughts about this aspect of audience may arise in considerations of the confidentiality of journals. Is someone quietly prying on a personal journal or not? If someone pries, does it matter? Is it all right that someone else learns more about one's views and reflections – more than would be revealed in a conversation? The coercion, the power and the nature of the audience can be major influences on journal writers and their journals.

Why write a learning journal?

There are many formal purposes (Moon, 1999b) for writing a journal (Chapter 5).

In this section we seek to provide a 'feel' for the reasons why people choose to engage in this activity. We tackle this task by considering the comments that journal writers and those who have managed a journal-writing process have made. These quotations are chosen because they seem, in their different ways, to articulate some of the essence of 'why write a journal'.

The personal journal has been used for hundreds of years to articulate the human drama of living and to explore new knowledge.

(Wolf, 1989)

Now I had a boyfriend and, without realizing why, I wrote that diary to and for him . . . One evening without fully understanding what I was doing, I suddenly scribbled across the page in a large hand: 'LET MY PAGE BE A WOMAN FOR THE FIRST TIME!' and then, 'There is nothing but blank before me. I don't know where to begin'. In that moment, on that page, I finally met myself as the audience of my own diary. In retrospect I consider it the single most important moment in my life.

(Rainer, 1978: 31)

The aim of the journal is partially to individualize the undergraduate psychology course. It is described to students as a means of connecting the knowledge, concepts and ideas which they acquire from the course to their past and present experiences, thoughts, work, self-reflections; books or articles read; and other courses.

(Hettich, 1976)

Keeping a Diary
I try to observe my own experience
And discover that the more I look the more I see
But I do not know how to learn from what I see.
(Joanna Field, 1952: 7)

[Journal-writing] . . . allows one to recognize, in writing, the natural thought processes.

(a student's comment in Wetherell and Mullins, 1996)

To some extent, we sense some meaning in each event as we live it. Much of the time, our response is so routine that the event adds little or nothing to our sense of our lives. Some events, though, carry a feeling of special meaning. Keeping a journal is another way in which we may grasp a fuller meaning in these events and in the situations in which we undergo them.

(Cell, 1984: 221)

The act of writing is a great stimulus to creativity. When we are grappling with a problem, it is a common occurrence that in writing down our conscious thoughts on the question, useful associations and new ideas begin to emerge. Writing the immediate thoughts makes more 'room' for new avenues of thinking, new possibilities.

(Miller, 1979)

How . . . [do] I learn . . . I wasn't really sure . . . Then, one summer, I discovered journals.

(Voss, 1988)

Education, as Frière noted rightly, can be used to free people or to domesticate them; when students write reflectively, I think they are being liberated.

(Sanford, 1988)

It is in the solitude of blank pages that adults can reflect on their life experiences, contemplate future directions, and come to trust more deeply in their own answers.

(Christensen, 1981)

Keeping a journal is a humbling process. You rely on your senses; your impressions and you purposely record your experiences as vividly, as playfully, and as creatively as you can. It is a learning process in which you are the learner and the one who teaches.

(Holly, 1991: 4)

The data, though not conclusive, seem to show that journals helped students clarify their thoughts and enhance their ability to develop ideas.

(Dimino, 1988 – of nursing students)

The purposes of the journal-writing assignments are to encourage exploration and risk-taking by the students as well as to teach content.

(Hahnemann, 1986)

I've learned that the private fingering of ordinary experience can fill up notebooks as interestingly as musings on great events . . . My own diaries have outgrown the green strongbox I used to keep them in, and I've outgrown believing that I'm such a shocking character that they need to be locked up. They're a permanent part of life now.

(Mallon, 1984)

I need to fill in the background . . . it centres on my diary. I have always written a diary – well – since I was around thirteen when I was given five-year diary for Christmas. That diary had a key and I used to hide the key inside a packet just inside the cover so I could slip it out. The diary saw me through the beginnings of my interests in boys and I was always worried that the diary would be read by my mother or by my young brother. I have gone on writing a diary. I suppose it has become part of me . . . something I just do. I usually write just before bedtime. My diary was first seriously challenged at uni. when my first boyfriend started to stay the night. Sitting side by side in a single bed

I could hardly say 'Sorry Martin, I want to write my diary. Just turn your head for a moment . . . would you.'

(Jaye, 2005 – from a short story)

The journal makes you more conscious of things – more aware. You think 'that would be useful to put in the journal' and then hold onto it. It 'highlights' things. It helps you to search for themes. It is useful to go back over your practice. You may not understand at first. You might annotate these things to think about ['unpack'] later. There may also be 'pop-up' issues – or issues in the news. The journal makes you notice things that might 'slip by'. I realise that I found the journal easier than other people. It is very different to academic work – a different way of working.

(From a student in Moon, 2004b)

In the concluding comments to his book, Hartley says: 'Finally . . . I would like to recommend some specific actions that learners might take to improve their learning and studying . . . to keep a reflective diary, making an entry at least once a week' (Hartley, 1998). This was a particularly important quotation in forming a conviction that there was a book to be written here! We have made no attempt here to distinguish the quotations that arise from journal work in formal educational or professional development settings from those that are personal. We have said that there is often not a clear dividing line between personal journals and those 'set' in a formal context.

The past and present contexts of learning journals

This section aims simply to set a context for the current popularity of learning journals with a brief review of past journal-writing and of its sources in more recent literature. By doing this we highlight the more influential voices of the field.

Lowenstein (1987) provides an excellent chronological account of journal-writing before this century. She mentions Japanese pillow books written by ladies of the court and the subsequent travel diaries written by Japanese travellers. These diaries at times shifted in their content between dream and fantasy and apparently objective truth. Many diaries have been written for spiritual or religious purposes, either as attempts to make sense of a person's relationship to deity or mankind, or they fulfil a more established role in the ritual. An example is the confessional diaries of the Puritans. Some diaries have had a deliberately community-building function, such as those of the Quakers, and many others relate to the records of lives or elements of lives lived which have been preserved for some reason where many others have been lost.

Mallon (1984) organizes another account of diary or journal-writing according to the apparent role of the diary in relation to the writer's life. In addition to travellers and confessors, he lists chroniclers, pilgrims, creators, apologists and prisoners. Under each of these headings, he explores many examples. A concluding comment from his studies is:

> After reading hundreds of diaries in the last several years, I've come to feel sure of three things. One is that writing books is too good an idea to be left to authors; another is that almost no one has had an easy life; and the third is that no one ever kept a diary for just himself.
>
> (Mallon, 1984)

A number of journal writers and designers of journals in more recent times seem to be closer, in their intentions for writing, to the notion of learning in learning journals. Tristine Rainer (1978) considers four of these to be of particular significance Carl Jung, Anais Nin, Joanna Field/Marion Milner (Field is a pen name) and Ira Progoff. These four pursued their journal-writing in different ways, in order that they could learn about themselves.

In the case of Jung, many of the discoveries that he made about himself were applied to his developing theories of psychology and psychotherapy. His book *Memories, Dreams and Reflections* comes close to being an autobiography, but at the same time is a rich record of personal learning, reasoning and reflection. In one incident, for example, from his adulthood, he describes the resolution of a period of personal tension. In trying to understand the underlying causes he decided to examine his past experiences and, failing to find explanation, 'I said to myself, "Since I know nothing at all, I shall do whatever occurs to me" ' (1961: 197). The first memory that appeared was of building miniature villages. He describes how he subjected himself to enacting the play again, making buildings with stones and mud, and as he did so, finding his mind clearing with 'the inner certainty that I was on the way to discovering my own myth' (1961: 198).

Marion Milner's writings are particularly interesting because, like Jung, she describes actions that she followed in pursuit of her understanding of herself. She describes her first book (Field, 1952), as 'a record of a seven years' study of living'. The aim of her study was to 'find out what kinds of experience made me happy' (1951: 13). The method she used was first to identify happy moments and to record them in detail and then to examine the records for patterns from which she could generalize. The book is written as a chronological account of the experiences and what she learns. The passage of her study took her well beyond only happy moments. For example, quite late on in the seven years, after experiences of disturbed feeling, she describes how she came to two conclusions:

> (i) The cause of any overshadowing burden of worry or resentment is never what it seems to be. Whenever it hangs over me like a cloud and refuses to disperse, then I must know that it comes from the area of blind thought and the real thing I am worrying about is hidden from me . . . (ii) To reason about such feelings, either in oneself or others, is futile.
>
> (Field, 1952: 140)

In another book, written a little later, Milner (now using her own name, and a practising psychoanalyst) records, in a similar way, a further personal project of learning to paint (Milner, 1957). Her meticulously recorded material on the four years of – what she called – an 'uncomfortable experience' led her to see painting as an interplay between objective and subjective views of the world: 'imagination and action, dream and reality, incorporated environment and external environment' (Milner, 1957: 129). This experience, she took further in her later explorations of personal functioning (e.g. Milner, 1987).

The work of Ira Progoff is similar to both in its active stance towards self-awareness and self-development using a journal (Progoff, 1975). Indeed, Progoff studied under Jung for some time. The format of the Intensive Journal consists of 19 named sections, into each of which different content is entered and across which there is extensive cross-referencing. As with Milner's work, there are extensive references to the Intensive Journal throughout this book, and it is described in more detail as an example of a journal in Chapter 12.

The work that Tristine Rainer herself did in developing 'the new diary' represents a very significant influence on journal-writing (Rainer, 1978). The 'new diary' draws from the work of previously mentioned writers and, particularly in contrast to Progoff, is very accessible and well organized. Rainer introduces seven techniques that she then applies to a variety of different human issues. The techniques include making lists, guided imagery, the use of dialogues and 'unsent letters'. Versions of these appear in Chapter 13. Examples of the issues to which these are applied are personal problems, the discovery of joy, work with dreams, exploring eroticism and so on. She makes a feature of the activity of rereading journal entries, which can become a source of new reflection and writing in itself. She points out that one never knows to where a diary will lead: 'One woman's diary began as a record of household expenses and expanded to a saga of her ancestors in the nineteenth century. One man's diary began as a punching-bag for his anger and became a haven where he opened up the poet and the songwriter in himself' (Rainer, 1978: 303).

Beyond these personally oriented writers about journal-writing, there are some more academic roots to journal-writing. Hettich has written about the use of journals with psychology students and learners in other disciplines (Hettich, 1976, 1980, 1988, 1990). In the early paper he refers to Allport's discussion of the uses of personal documents as a method of research. Allport himself is clearly impressed with the data that can enter journals: 'The spontaneous, intimate diary is the personal document par excellence . . . In its ideal form the diary is unexcelled as a continuous record of the subjective side of mental development' (Allport, 1942: 95).

In the mid-1980s Holly picked up on another increasingly important use of journal-writing in the context of professional development, in particular teacher education. Holly's book, which is found in a number of editions (e.g. Holly, 1991), is a succinct and 'down to earth' gathering of information written alongside a large literature of other discussions of the use of journals in this field.

Another root from which journal-writing has developed, particularly in the United States, is from the proponents of writing as a means of learning. There are many ways in which writing can be linked to learning and the enhancement of learning and memory, and this reasoning has been used to advance the cause of journal-writing (Britton, 1972; Emig, 1977; Elbow, 1981; Yinger and Clark, 1981). This constitutes some of the subject matter of Chapters 2 and 3. Emerging from this line of thinking were two books in the mid-1980s that probably represent the best source material for ideas and methods of journal-writing. The first, edited by Young and Fulwiler (1986), is a collection of papers about the value of writing of different forms in all disciplines. The second is also an edited collection of articles on the use of journals in all areas of the college curriculum (Fulwiler, 1987).

One more root of journal work should be mentioned because it is certainly playing a very significant part in sustaining and building the use of journals at present. It is the development of the theory and practice of reflection itself. The work of four writers tends to be particularly associated with theories of reflection in a fundamental manner. The first two are more theory-based. Dewey (1933) views reflection as an acute thinker/observer and interprets his observations from an educational standpoint. Habermas (1971) is an epistemologist and for him, the role of reflection is as a tool in the development of different forms of human knowledge. Schön (1983, 1987) instigated the wide use of the term 'the reflective practitioner'. Kolb came from the traditions of experiential learning. The Kolb cycle of experiential learning (Kolb, 1984) identifies reflection as one stage of learning and is sometimes used to structure journal work (e.g. Wolf, 1980). In addition, we should add the contribution to reflection of the book of Boud *et al.* (1985), *Reflection: Turning Experience into Learning*, which itself was broadly based on Kolb's work.

In practical terms, as we have mentioned earlier, the work on reflection has expanded greatly across higher education in the UK as institutions have addressed the need to put into place some form of reflective activity that relates a student's learning experience to future planning and career development. This is termed 'personal development profiling, or planning' (PDP) and sometimes the term 'professional development planning' is used in professional contexts (Chapter 6).

In terms of current developments of the use of learning journals, we cannot ignore the role of the electronic screen. We now have blogs and wikis. Some would extol the virtues of these forms as beyond anything that we have had before in any other format – perhaps they are those who have never, themselves, used the pen and paper version of personal journals. In the end it is the human being and the products of the human mind that makes the journal work or not work – not the nature of paper or screen on which the ideas are scrolled . . . And this even applies to the *Big Brother* 'diary room' (Channel 4, 2005)!

We noted in the first edition of this book that more seemed (at the time) to be written about journals in teacher and nurse education than in any other form of higher education, and further that the use of journals in these forms of professional education is often related to their adoption of 'reflective practice'. There is certainly still considerable use of journals in these two professions, but their use, often justified by the notion of developing 'the reflective practitioner' is much more widespread now – though what exactly is meant by 'reflective practice' is still idiosyncratic (Moon, 2004a). The speculation, in the first edition, about why it should be that journals are common in teaching and nursing still stands – reflective learning and the use of journals tends to be more broadly associated with the female gender.

The personal origins of this book on learning journals

It is becoming usual for writers to tell the story of how they came to write a book (e.g. Boud and Miller, 1996). In this book such a practice is further justified in a manner that represents some of the reasoning behind the writing of journals. Our perception of the world is based on the set of experiences of which we have been a part. Since we then further interpret the world through those perceptions, it is useful for a reader to understand some autobiographical influences on the product of a writer's mind.

I begin . . . (we are now clearly in the realm of the first person singular) settling now into a style of writing that comes from many, many years of writing journals. As in Weil, (1996) the letter, 'I' seems to be a trigger to set me into this writing style.

I began writing diaries when I was 11 years old. Looking at the tatty red note-book, it seems that I mainly wrote only on holidays to begin with. The entries are notes about what we did as a family – usually about swimming and sometimes deteriorating to days described lazily as – 'as usual'. There are no reflective accounts at this stage, though I know that my daughter at the age of 11 was capable of deeply reflective personal writing. Alongside my diary of that time, though, I have another notebook, this covered in plastic kitchen tablecloth with bottles and wine glasses on it. It is a story I wrote when I was about 12. It did not start out to be autobiographical, but I know that that is how it became. It explored the depths of feelings of that age and I think that that is where I truly began to reflect. It was easier, at first, to displace my musings into fiction. The story certainly seems to belong with my diaries. We explore the role of story in journals in Chapter 11.

The next diary is a locking five-year diary in green. My current self does not know where the key is and I wonder if I will have to break in this time, but I find that my hands feel for the tag and I watch them pull out the key. They clearly know more than I do. Pulling out the key is a habit of all those five years because there is five years' worth of close handwriting – my adolescence in 5×365 entries, beginning at the age of 14. I can now see reflectivity creeping in 'School was very much as usual today, but I was very much teased about liking Chris Collins (and I do). I wonder if he likes me . . .' Flicking further through the pages I come to an encoded area and I am pleased to find a list of the codes. Adolescence must have its secrets (adolescence alone, I query?). The information that I had been kissed for the first time was too sensitive to be displayed in readable text, even in a locked diary. Thinking about my mother's horror of two years later when she learned that I might have been kissing with a boy leads me to think, even now, that there was justification for the code, if not the lock as well.

I open the red lockable five-year diary, which covers the period from age 19 to 23. I glance through the entries. There is one about going to a restaurant. I wrote what I ate. I recall that meal. It was a windy and wet night. Without my writing of the time, it is unlikely that that experience would ever have emerged again. I notice another entry, this time on my 23rd birthday. John was my husband – the marriage did not last. I wrote:

> John gave me (as an extra) a box of mint creams and a box of chocolates – I cannot imagine why – I cannot bear sweets for presents and wish he'd learn. I expect he'll eat most of them anyway. He keeps me neatly in stock and eats most of the sweets himself. I think it is mean and disappointing.

I do not suppose that I ever quietly conveyed my resentment to the poor man. If this were a true learning journal, I would like to think that I would have intended to take action rather than simply observing.

The third five-year diary took me out of the marriage and into what I have always felt was my true adolescence. The diary is not complete. In June 1975 it stops abruptly because I attended a Progoff Intensive Journal Workshop in Edinburgh and began an entirely different form of writing. Attending the workshop that weekend influenced my life and, in itself, was a profound experience for the spiritual feelings that were generated by working with a group of people in that manner.

The example in Chapter 12 provides more information about the Intensive Journal. I have mentioned the 19 sections above. In my bookcases, I have three or four fat tomes of loose-leaf pages in the 19 sections. From early on, though, the entries in the daily log predominated, often expanding into manners of working that should have been cross-referenced and placed in other sections. For long-term and day-to-day working, I have always felt that the Intensive Journal is too complex for long-term use for those with busy family and working lives and that is why I have considered how it might be made easier to use. For short periods of time or for workshops, I think that the structure is very facilitative and powerful. On the basis of these thoughts, which have come to a head in tackling journal-writing in objective terms in this book, I have redesigned the journal that I keep. I describe the new format in Chapter 12 as an example of how to keep a journal.

Over the years I believe that there were one or maybe two gaps during which I did not write for a time. I almost certainly wrote the equivalent material into letters to friends even if I did not retain a record of it. I have never chosen to share what I have written in journals. In one or two places among the pages of journals there are (loose) notes for the attention of others whom I knew, at the time, to be peeping. I feel a sense of intrusion when this has happened. On one occasion, at the bad end of a relationship, I faked a few entries, implying that I was having another relationship. Sure enough, the issue of this 'affair' arose in flames and the culprit truly indicted himself. The lesson I learnt from that, though, was how difficult it was to extricate myself from my act of fiction. He would not believe that my entries were not genuine! In the last year, I have incorporated the experience of this interesting episode into real fiction in a short story – and in so doing have learnt much more (Jaye, 2005). Journals and story are closely related (Chapter 11).

I come to the present. My 'brief' journal lies on the table in front of me, a small flat folder covered with red leather, which fits into my handbag. The brief, portable version of the journal feeds pages into a larger non-portable version – long-live loose leaf when it comes to journals! – and I will come back to this later. I have become more conscious of the learning aspect of journal-writing as I have read papers in preparation for this book. I enjoy noticing when I learn something new about myself. From that point of view, I have great admiration for the sustained learning projects of Joanna Field (Marion Milner). One day, when there is more time . . .

This leads me to the last paragraphs before I pull back into more objective language. How has journal-writing affected me and how has it contributed to my life? A journal is a friend that is always there and is always a comfort. In bad moments, I write, and usually end up feeling better. It reflects back to me things that I can learn about my world and myself. It represents a private space in my life, a beautiful solitude, the moments before I go to sleep just to stop and note what is 'there' about the day or about my life at the time. I think that it has enabled me to feel deeper and more established as a person, more in control but more trusting of life. On a less introverted note, I think that it contributes to my ability to write in general, and it underlies an interest in poetry and creative writing largely which also awaits a quieter time in my life for fulfilment. In addition, I consider that journal-writing is closely linked with the counselling and hypnotherapy work that I have done over the years. It has been a support and a resource and a means of exploration, though I cannot say whether journal-writing led to counselling or whether they both emerged as a result of particular traits in my personality.

The contributions from journal-writing to my life have not come about through one or two entries to a journal. They have come over a long time. This represents a very important area of learning for me, the truth of which has only dawned as I have spoken with others who write journals. My view of the world, even what I learn from what I write in any one entry, is not 'truth'. It represents my construct of what appears to be truth in that moment and in another moment the learning may be different. Alongside the learning from the making of any one entry, I need to have the ability to put judgement on hold and watch how subsequent entries shape the same issue. That is when the universality of the learning becomes evident – or not.

Now I need to reflect a little on how I am as I arrive at the stool in front of the computer writing this second edition. I have written three books since the first edition – one of which is of key importance to this. It is a revisiting of reflective learning which feeds into the rewriting of this (Moon, 2004a). For seven years I have also run workshops in the UK and abroad on reflective learning and learning journals (and other things). This means that thousands of people have come, listened and discussed their experiences and needs and interests. I cannot but be influenced by what I have heard. A particular issue that comes up at workshops that needs to be incorporated into this edition of the book is on ethical issues and journal-writing. I realized its importance when a participant said that her department had abandoned the use of journals (in a professional education context) because the ethical issues were too extreme to be managed.

After seven years I remain passionate about journal-writing as a creative and developmental process and the first edition of this book was the book that I enjoyed writing more than any other. One day there will be a non-academic version of it and there will be non-academic/community-based workshops on the use of learning journals too. In terms of my interests, I feel I have come to understand much more about learning and that understanding is written into the first chapters of the 2004 book. I had to relate reflection to learning – as few others have engaged in exploring this link and it seems crucial to the role of reflection in higher education. Recently I set out to explore critical thinking in higher education. I have long considered this term to be intriguing because it is both central to higher education and yet its nature and processes are vague. The paper that resulted both drew from my work on reflection and has contributed to it – and references to it will be represented in this book (Moon, 2005a). I have also become more interested in story and the role of fiction in our lives. This interest is represented in a little writing of short stories and poetry and in particular in the act of oral storytelling – and it has inspired the addition of Chapter 11 to this edition. None of it feels far from meaningful forms of formal education or from journal-writing.

The layout of this book

This chapter has introduced the idea of learning journals and some reasons why this book came to be written. While this chapter has already begun to use the term 'learning journal', it is Chapter 2 that seeks the justification for the name. How do journals help learning? We consider some of the underpinning theory of learning and of representing that learning in writing that relates to the practice of journal-writing. The chapter contains new material for the second edition and there is now a third chapter – perhaps the part of the book that most needed revision since the work in Moon (2004a). It develops ideas of depth and quality of reflection assuming that superficial reflection leads to superficial learning. We want to ensure, therefore, that students reflect with more depth.

Chapter 5 explores the surprisingly wide range of purposes for which journals are employed both personally and in educational situations. Chapter 6 is concerned with the application of learning journals in many disciplines in higher education. The expectation might well be that learning journals only have a place in the humanities or other disciplinary areas in which sustained writing is a normal practice. In fact the literature provides accounts of the use of journals in over 30 disciplines and these are probably sufficient to allow us the suggestion that learning journals have potential application in any subject matter.

Despite the wide range of literature about journals in disciplinary contexts, the greater volume of literature probably seems to come from their use in professional development, particularly in teacher education programmes. Chapter 7 considers their role in these subject areas – in initial and continuing professional development, in institutional contexts and in the context of short courses. Although it may be difficult to separate personal from professional development, some accounts of the use of journals clearly relate only to the personal element, to which Chapter 8 is devoted. This chapter is considerably expanded to include reference to personal development planning in higher education (PDP).

Chapter 9 is practical and is concerned with the 'how to' issues: it discusses the format of journals; problems of starting to write; how to help those who seem to find reflection difficult; the conditions for successfully sustaining the writing of journals and so on. This chapter is considerably revised in the second edition, adding material on how to get students started with reflection. Chapter 10 takes on the difficult topic of the assessment of learning journals and again is now considerably revised because, since the first book was written, the author has changed her mind about the assessment of journals. While it may not always be necessary to assess reflective work, in many situations in higher education, journals would simply not be kept if there were not some form of assessment process associated with the activity. The chapter provides practical guidance on this matter.

Chapter 11 is a new chapter for the new edition and it concerns the role of story in journal-writing, both to enrich the process of writing journals, to link it with the world of imagination and creativity and to draw in another interesting area of literature. Chapter 12 provides examples of different kinds of journals that might be kept under different circumstances and an expanded Chapter 13 provides a range of activities that are useful in the process of journal-writing.

We end this chapter, as indeed, we will end all chapters, with another quotation. It is not unusual to open a chapter with a quotation – but personal experience suggests that at the beginning of a chapter, the reader may be anxious to get on with the chapter. We add the quotations at the end of the chapter in the spirit of the journal – leaving the reader with something about which to think. The quotations are selected for their illustration of the rich experience of journal-writing.

Thinkpoint

A reflection on the calendar from Edith Holden's *The Country Diary of an Edwardian Lady*

This month received its present name from the Emperor Augustus, and was selected, not as being his natal month, but because in it his greatest fortune happened to him. As July contained 31 days, it was thought necessary to add another day to the latter month in order that Augustus might not be in any respect inferior to Julius.

(Holden, 1977: 106)

Chapter 2

Learning from learning journals

Journals and the process of learning

Introduction

One of the main criteria for the 'learning journal' is that there is an intention to learn from it, though we recognize that early attempts at journal-writing, even in an academic context, are often very descriptive. The learning from descriptive writing might seem to represent a different quality of learning from that which occurs when a person writes reflectively. Reflective writing could be likened to using the page as a meeting place in which ideas can intermingle and, in developing, give rise to new ideas for new learning. The 'thinkpoint' quotation at the end of this chapter is an illustration of this point.

There is no one type of learning that results from working with journals but in saying that we make no excuses for the seeming dearth of material that relates the use of journals to the learning process – learning from the journal process seems to be assumed. McCrindle and Christensen (1995) and Dart *et al.* (1998) represent exceptions to this in their concern for the wider consequences for learning of using a learning journal.

In this book we deal with the issue of how students learn from journals by taking two angles on the topic. In this chapter we consider the broader issues of how students learn, and relate this to reflective learning and, of course, the learning from journals. This is a chapter that some readers may wish to leave out in their first consideration of the topic of learning journals. In the next chapter – still on learning, we look at the manner in which journal-writing enables or encourages learning through favouring the conditions that are recognized to enhance learning. The coverage of the relationship of learning to reflection and reflective writing is a condensed and abbreviated version of that in Moon (2004a).

Learning, reflection and learning journals

There are many areas of theory about learning that can inform our understanding of how students learn from learning journals. The bodies of theory are not completely separated, nor is there consistency within them. For example, those who write on reflection as a topic come from different origins or disciplines, and tend not to have gone far outside their own field of research on the literature. As a consequence those who write about reflection in journals bring a very broad literature and multiple interpretations. It seems that often writers cannot make sense of the whole field in a few introductory paragraphs and grasp one or two significant names and base their discussion on those names. In reviewing the work on reflection in previous books (Moon, 1999a, 2004a), it has seemed that Dewey (1933), Schön (1983, 1987) and Boud *et al.* (1985) are key figures in the history of the topic.

Beyond reflection, a further concept of 'reflective practice' has come into greater use, with learning journals often being the tool used to facilitate its development. It is a term that is vague in meaning but broadly seems to imply that a person is active in reflecting on events and using what she can learn from them to improve future action. There is now an Institute for Reflective Practice (Institute of Reflective Practice, 2005) that has facilitates learning about reflection, and disseminates ideas via conferences. It publishes journal in which there are many papers on learning journals (*Journal of Reflective Practice*).

How students learn: with a focus on learning from journal processes

To begin with there are a few points to be made about learning:

- The learning to which this section refers is not the learning of physical skills, but other learning that is deliberate, is probably organized and in many contexts, and is formal.
- Emotion is considered to be involved in all learning (this point is addressed in the Chapter 3).
- We are talking about learning here and not teaching. Teaching and learning are different. Learners learn but teachers teach and try to facilitate learners' learning, but what a teacher teaches may not be what is learnt by the learner. For convenient differentiation, we introduce two new terms: 'material of teaching' – what a teacher teaches, and 'material of learning' – what a learner learns.
- We can only assess the learning of a person through the representation of her learning – in written, spoken, or graphic form (etc.). The representation of learning is not the initial learning itself but a secondarily processed version of it – and it is this secondary version that goes into a journal. People may be more proficient at one form of representation than another (e.g. more proficient at oral rather than written representation).
- We learn from the process of representing learning (Eisner, 1991) – we learn also from the process of representing the initial learning in a journal (as a secondary process).

Some basic ideas about learning

We start by distinguishing between two stances on learning. The first stance is the popular conception of learning – the accumulation model of learning. In this model, knowledge is 'taken in' and it builds up as if a brick wall were being built. A teacher may be seen as the supplier of the bricks of knowledge and in this role, she needs to know what the learner knows in order to lay the correct blocks of knowledge. If the learner realizes that she has some incorrect knowledge, she replaces the one 'brick' of knowledge with another. This is the conception of learning that forms the basis of most popular language about learning. It could relate to descriptive writing in journals – but not writing that has depth.

The second stance on learning is the constructivist view. It suggests that, instead of a brick wall, the metaphor for knowledge is a flexible network of ideas and feelings; some closely associated and some much further apart. Some ideas have few links in the network; some are heavily interconnected. The term 'cognitive structure' tends to be used to describe this notional network (West and Pines, 1985; McAlpine and Weston, 2002). This is the model that best supports the idea of good journal learning.

On the constructivist view, new material of learning (e.g. a new idea) is linked into the network, but in being linked in, it may be modified in the process of assimilation (Piaget, 1971). As new ideas are linked in, they may cause change in the cognitive structure itself – the process of accommodation (Piaget, 1971). We have now moved beyond the simple idea of accumulation of knowledge to the more flexible idea that the material of learning and the existing knowledge (cognitive structure) may change in the process of learning. The process of writing a journal may often be the playing out of this activity with paper and pen – 'how does this new idea/or experience relate to what I thought I knew?'

There are two important ideas here. First, the cognitive structure may change without the addition of new material of learning. We 'change our minds'. There is no new material of learning. This closely accords with the notion of reflection in a learning journal. Second, the state of the cognitive structure guides the process of assimilation – in other words, what we learn is guided by what we already know. It is not guided by what the teacher thinks the learner knows – but by what the learner does know (or knows that she does not know). It is the sense that the learner makes of material of learning that is important. Again, on the basis of this, learning is not accumulation, but a process of changing one's conceptions – or, ultimately, of transforming oneself. A journal may play a part in helping a learner to clarify for herself what she does know about something in order that she can understand new material of learning (e.g. in the next lecture).

Some features of the process of accommodation

Learning is a matter of relating and balancing existing knowledge and new material of learning – but other factors will come in as well. For example, a highly motivated learner on a short course, who trusts the material of teaching and knows that the new material of learning can be of benefit to her, may allow a complete change of her cognitive structure in response to the material of teaching. However, another learner, who was sent on a course and is an unwilling learner, or who may have little trust in the material of teaching, may either not pay attention or may use other areas of her cognitive structure to construct arguments that reject the new material of learning (e.g. 'I know this already'). Most of what we learn formally is relatively in accordance with our expectations and that facilitates the processes of assimilation and accommodation. Sometimes, however, we learn something that demands considerable changes in our systems of knowledge and belief and we might initially reject the material (a good example here would be a challenge to religious beliefs). Later, change might start to occur, but it can take time for all the various understandings to become consistent. Changes in associated actions may take even longer (e.g. change in political belief may mean that there is need for a change in social behaviour as well). Cognitive dissonance is a term for the situation in which there is conflict between current knowledge and new material of learning (Festinger, 1957). It can be uncomfortable and may often be a process explored in journals.

The last few paragraphs have much to do with the use of learning journals. A journal may be a place for exploring the degree to which a learner 'trusts' material of teaching or her expectations in relation to new material of learning and a journal may be used to support subsequent change. This is a strong justification for the use of journals to support professional education and development (e.g. Brookfield, 1995; Tsang, 2003) or to support those who are entering situations in which their beliefs may be challenged (Trelfa, 2005; Moon, 2004a). Journals very often will be used to support the exploration of the meaningfulness of an idea – but what does 'meaning' mean?

What is 'meaningfulness'?

Ausubel and Robinson (1969) believed in meaningfulness as a quality of the material of teaching – saying that the teacher decides what are meaningful concepts. Unintentionally, however, they supported the case that meaningfulness is a quality attributed to the material by the individual learner. In an example, they suggested that a three-letter unit – 'LUD' is meaningless. Anyone who knows British comedy television, would be likely to have a meaning for 'lud' in the phrase 'yes, me lud' (i.e. 'yes, my Lord' – a phrase that might be used in a court scene). We suggest that the attribution of meaning is primarily a task for the learner. The same idea can legitimately be meaningful to one learner and not to another – because of different prior experiences. There are, of course, social issues about meaning. We agree on many meanings or we could not live in communities. However, it is important for the idea of learning, that we recognize that meaning is first a matter for the individual since the learner makes sense of ideas for herself. However, the tools and practices that operate in the process of making sense have been developed as a social process (Lave and Wenger, 1991; Wilkes, 1997). Children do not learn everything from 'new', but use the cultural accumulation of ideas in order to interpret the world. Language is a socially developed tool. Where there is not a word for something, the idea does not usually exist in public terms – hence, for example, the need to develop new words to describe learning and teaching (see above on 'material' of learning and teaching). However, obviously and less obviously, cultures of understanding differ – e.g. different disciplines, different religions, different politics and different nationalities manage and use knowledge differently. This has proved to be an issue in the introduction of reflective learning and journals to students whose first language and culture is that of the educational system (e.g. Stockhausen and Kawashima, 2002). There is not always a word for 'reflection' in a national language.

Learning and experience

The use of journals is often justified by the need to help students to learn from their experiences (e.g. in a placement) – and hence it is important to explore the process of learning from experience. In effect, all learning is learning from experience. Sometimes the experience is mediated. By 'mediated', we mean that it is manipulated, interpreted, simplified and reorganized into what is probably a more comprehensible sequence for a learner – a teacher mediates. Mediated experience is still experience even if part of the experience is that of sitting in a lecture theatre, and another bit of the experience is the voice of the lecturer and the meanings that the material stimulates in the learner. In other words, we suggest that 'experiential learning' is not really 'special' in the manner in which it is often treated (for more discussion on this matter, see Moon 2004a).

We illustrate issues in experience and learning through a scenario. We have said that we build meanings by working with experience. We learn (something) in relationship to our present and prior experience since the prior experience (i.e. the state of the cognitive structure) guides how we respond to a present experience. We have said that the nature of experience is individual in the sense that it is an individual who experiences it, but social, in that all experience is mediated by the social surroundings. In the scenario, there is a field trip in one module for adult students on a Geology course. Readers might imagine the kinds of entries that Alice (see below) makes in a journal that covers this module. (In this section some of the material is direct quotation from Moon (2004).)

There is a type of limestone quarried at Beer in Devon (UK) that has long been valued because it is easy to quarry and to saw into shape. In the open atmosphere it hardens to form an excellent building stone. It has been used for construction of many major buildings. A learner, Alice, in an adult and continuing education programme, sees on the web that that she will be going on a field trip to Beer to visit the underground quarries and to learn about the geology of the site. She has not heard of Beer or of Beer stone at first. Beer is a word and a place. The word might initially trigger associations with the drink, but this link will probably fade away as the meaningfulness of Beer as a place gains ascendancy. The notion of Beer stone might be meaningless at present – but is likely, having been listed in the curriculum, to be potentially meaningful to the learner when she relates it to other types of stone that she has studied. A male colleague, Georgio, another learner who is also going on the trip, went to Beer while on holiday last year and saw the quarries. As a result he has a cognitive structure that enables the concept (of Beer stone) to be meaningful. The meaning might be associated with seeing the material but also with the stories told of the history of the quarrymen on a guided trip round the quarries. His meaning for 'Beer' will, in some measure, be directly shaped by social means in the form of the accounts told by the guide.

Before the trip Alice asks Georgio about Beer and Georgio expresses his learning in the form of a story about the stone – its appearance and texture but also the memories that he has of the signatures of the seventeenth-century quarrymen that he has seen on the walls of the quarries. The story is socially constructed and triggers prior experiences in the mind of Alice (e.g. of once, with a boyfriend of adolescent years, trying to inscribe their linked names on a slab of limestone). Eventually there is a lecture on the course that includes reference to the chemistry and geological origins of this limestone that gives rise to its qualities. We note that the study of limestone could be part of biology – in that it is developed from biological material (shells), or maritime studies (since it was formed under the sea), or engineering because it is a construction material – and so on. The fact that the ideas are being covered in geology means that any investigation in a practical sense will be geological, and any reports written will have used geological termin-ology. Geology, like other disciplines, is a human construction in itself, and influences the structure of what we know.

Eventually Alice and Georgio and the other learners go on the field trip and see, touch and in other ways experience Beer stone. Alice can accommodate her prior knowledge (gained from her conversations with Georgio) to the new and personal experiences of the stone. The concept of Beer stone might then said to be more meaningful to her. Her journal might have 'logged' the way in which the meaning has been constructed.

The paragraphs above illustrate the social nature of learning and knowledge and how the learning process itself is socially mediated. Before the lecture on Beer stone from her conversation with Georgio, Alice had a number of experiences that created a 'slot' for the meaning of Beer stone in her cognitive structure which was represented by a set of expectations. These prior experiences are likely to have influenced the manner in which she received the new information. For example, if she was told in the lecture that a feature of the stone is that it is so hard that it cannot be scratched, she would have material to re-evaluate (e.g. was Georgio's story credible when he told her about the quarrymen's signatures? Was he talking about some other stone? Is the lecturer credible?). There would be cognitive dissonance which might be disturbing – but again that could be usefully explored in the form of a journal.

External and internal experience – and meaning

It is useful to introduce the terminology 'external' and 'internal' experience at this point (Marton and Booth, 1997). External experience is the material of learning when we are learning about something that is generally outside of ourselves. It is the object, idea, the concept, the image – whatever it is that the learner wants to assimilate. In contrast, the internal experience is the experience that the learner brings to the learning situation from her current cognitive structure. It is the sum of prior experiences (knowledge of, feelings about) the object.

Before her visit to Beer and sight of the stone, Alice built up an internal mental experience which was to do with scratch-ability, chemical and geological qualities as well as the story of quarrying processes and so on. When she saw the rock, the learning process involved the interaction or flux between these forms of experience in order to develop her own new perspective. This again is a process that may be worked out in its form of written representation in the journal.

The passage below describes another aspect of meaning. Meaning changes with experience of a particular object, but it may change with alterations in the experience of other objects that are related to the first object. We return to the experiences of Alice: later in her programme, after her visit to Beer, Alice might learn more about the chemistry involved in the fossilization process. Beer stone, itself, might not have been mentioned in the lecture on fossilization, but her broader knowledge about stone and fossilization will invest more and possibly different meanings in the concept of Beer stone. We mentioned how thinking about Beer stone in buildings could also lead to an enriched concept. There might be, however, different qualities of meaning: on the field trip, someone jokes that Beer stone is, of course, hardened by painting beer on it. This too can become part of the 'meaning' of Beer stone – a meaning that might be exploited again in humour, or myth, or in writing a story.

The frame of reference of an experience will determine the distinction of the figure from the ground (what we need to attend to and what we reject in a particular context). For example, if the students are told that the field trip is for the purpose of gaining knowledge of the history of quarrying, the art and history of the stone is not going to be relevant to the field trip. We use our internal experience and guidance from others, if it is available, in order to distinguish what we need to learn from what is not needed for the current sense-making.

Meaning is not present or absent but something that is invested in a person's internal experience of an object. When interpreting or representing meaning, the learner will try to pull out the meaning relevant to the context. A poem relating to the East Devon coast might pull out very different meanings of Beer stone to those meanings with which the learner works in an examination question about the geology of limestone – but they are all meanings of Beer stone to a particular individual.

To learn something, we also need to be able to be clear what it is we want to learn and to distinguish it from other distractions – we can use the concept of the distinction of figure from ground to describe this process. Looking at the Beer stone, it is important to be able to access the relevant internal experience of the stone at a particular time which is pertinent to the current preoccupation.

Journals and learning

This is all rich ground for learning from learning journals. Writing a journal enables a learner to go back over material that she has learned and expand the ideas or the linkages between ideas in relation to the original learning, explore internal experience (the sum of prior experiences), the way in which external experience relates to internal experience, how the 'meaning' of an event or an object to one person is related to that meaning for the writer – and so on. The journal is also a place for self explanations that arise in making sense of something (Chi *et al.* 1989, 1994). In terms of the concept of frame of reference and the distinction of figure from ground, the learner's perspective on any stated purpose for a learning journal will be important as well as her understanding of what is meant by the act of reflective writing. The distinction from figure and ground can be a central purpose of writing in a learning journal, when, for example, we are exploring an issue and trying to find the aspects of it on which we need or wish to focus. While in formal writing such as an essay, the 'track' of the flow of meaning though the text is within strict boundaries, in a journal there is freedom to explore.

The ability to focus appropriately on the object of reflection (i.e. distinguishing figure from ground) is very relevant to the distinction of reflective writing of a descriptive and of a deeper level (see Chapter 4). In the latter there is more clarity about the focus of the reflection.

A brief summary and a few more points

We have said that we learn through the assimilation of material of learning and accommodation of the cognitive structure. Generally when there is information external to the person, the material of learning is conceived as an external experience. We learn through the comparison of external experience with the current internal experiences that we bring to bear on the material of learning. Internal experience is the relevant prior knowledge and experience that guides the means of assimilation through guiding our frames of reference in relation to external experience. This enables us to focus on the relevant variations in the current external experience and to take account of the variations between current internal and external experience. In the process of assimilating new material of learning the cognitive structure accommodates. We talk of conceptions being changed or transformed in the process of learning. In learning, these processes operate in at least two ways – learning about content and also learning about learning. As a learner progresses, in other words, becomes a more efficient learner, she learns more content, but she also learns more about learning.

On the basis of this model, we see reflective learning initially as the kind of learning that occurs when there is no new material of learning. We have suggested that in this context it is best conceived as a process of reordering of internal experience (Moon, 2004a), coining the term 'cognitive housekeeping' to provide metaphorical meaning. We have suggested that reflection may sometimes occur when there is new material of learning that is ill-structured or complex and where the learner intends to understand meaningfully. In these situations reflection seems to accord with the functioning of internal experience, relating what is known to the new material. We might also reflect when we learn from the representation of learning – in other words, when we write (etc.) something down and then what we have written stimulates more thinking (and perhaps redrafting).

Learning about learning can be conceived as taking place along the same lines as learning about content. There is the operation of frames of reference that focus the learner on tasks of the learning process, with the importance of the distinction of figure from ground and with the variation between internal and external experience being the stimulus to learn. This process may be practised in a journal or the subject matter of the journal-writing.

Thinkpoint

Harry . . . [stared] at the stone basin. The contents had returned to their original, silvery white state, swirling and rippling beneath his gaze.

'What is it?' Harry asked shakily.

'This? It is called a Pensieve,' said Dumbledore. 'I sometimes find, and I am sure that you know the feeling, that I simply have too many thoughts and memories crammed into my mind.'

'Er,' said Harry, who couldn't truthfully say that he had ever felt anything of the sort.

'At these times,' said Dumbledore, indicating the stone basin, 'I use the Pensieve. One simply siphons the excess thoughts from one's mind, pours them into the basin, and examines them at one's leisure. It becomes easier to spot patterns and links, you understand, when they are in this form.'

(Rowling, 2000: 518–19)

Chapter 3

How students learn from learning journals

Journal-writing as a process that accentuates favourable conditions for learning

Introduction

In the previous chapter we explored some of the relationships between learning, reflection and journal-writing. We were able to show how reflection is part of the process of learning, and how writing a journal can enhance both, within a mutually reinforcing system. Journals also accentuate the favourable conditions for learning, affecting learning in a range of less direct manners. There are a number of ways in which this occurs and we explore these in the course of this chapter. There are many types of journals, many purposes, many forms – hence the need to generalize. In enhancing the favourable conditions for learning, journal-writing:

- slows the pace of learning
- can increase the sense of ownership of learning
- acknowledges the role of emotion in learning
- give learners an experience of dealing with ill-structured material of learning
- encourages metacognition (learning about one's own process of learning)
- enhances learning through the process of writing.

These issues are explored in this chapter.

Journals slow the pace of learning

Journal-writing that is reasonably adept favours learning by demanding time and 'intellectual space' (Barnett, 1997). The learner is forced to stop and think in order to write and in an educational or professional environment, such time for reflection or writing can be difficult to achieve by other means (Walker, 1985; Wildman and Niles, 1987). Lack of time, of course, is a reason why journal-writing can fail (Selfe and Arbabi, 1986).

When we talk about the notions of time and intellectual space, we should not forget the closely related quality of silence. The writing of a journal gives an opportunity to develop that quality of 'contemplative silence' that Dawson suggests 'nourishes the creative impulse lying at the heart of all significant learning and living' (Dawson, 2003). Alerby and Elidottir (2003) explore the notions of silence with regard to reflection. They end on the note: 'In the process of reflection, silence can be observed as a sense-making process which emphasises learning in, with and through silence. It is important to listen to and be with others, but also to listen to ourselves, understand and value the sounds of silence and use its many melodies' (Alerby and Elidottir, 2003). From the experiences of the writer, there is a very special quality of the silence that occurs when a roomful of people are engaged in the reflective writing of a learning journal.

In that time–space in which learners write in their journals, they are, by the definition of the activity, undergoing independent learning and the encouragement of independent thought is a means of enhancing learning. The learners are forced to be self-sufficient because there is no specific answer to any question that they might ask about 'what shall I write?', though there may be structures or questions that will prompt their writing. To the degree that journal-writing is independent, it is also 'owned' by the writer.

Journals increase the sense of ownership of learning

Although content of a journal may be within provided guidelines, the essential nature of journal-writing means that – to use a metaphor – the writer is at the wheel and is steering. Rogers suggests that 'significant learning takes place when the subject matter is perceived by the student as having relevance for his own purpose' (1969: 158). For the writer, the writing of a journal provides a focusing point, an opportunity to order thoughts (engage in 'cognitive housekeeping', see Chapter 2) and to make sense of a situation or of information. In training courses, even of one day, an opportunity to write reflectively can enable participants to 'collect their thoughts' about a matter that has been discussed with a variety of opinions aired. They can relate the new material of learning to their own experiences or previous knowledge (i.e. an internal experience, see Chapter 2). The nature of the learning, once reinforced by a journal, is likely to be more robust.

Journals acknowledge the role of emotion in learning

Most, though not all, uses of journals involve the acknowledgement or the expression of emotion which is considered to be a more complete form of learning (Boud et al., 1985). Rogers says: 'Self initiated learning which involves the whole persona of the learner – feelings as well as intellect – is the most lasting and pervasive . . . This is not learning that takes place "only from the neck-up". It is a gut-level type of learning . . .' (Rogers, 1969: 163).

It is clear that the topic of emotion surrounds the use of journals. Field (1952) tried to learn about her own behaviour initially by observing what made her happy. Storr (1988) provides examples of how a number of writers appear to have used autobiographical writing as a means of coping with or working through the emotional deprivations of their childhoods. He applies this principle, with reference to journal-writing, to Beatrix Potter. Rainer (1978) quotes a vivid emotional passage from 'one diarist': 'I feel the pain which has been forcing itself to the surface for the past four months. It swells inside me like a huge egg pushing its way out of my throat . . . I write here in the diary, hoping that I will be delivered of this pain' (Rainer, 1978: 116–17).

Emotion seems to have many different relationships to reflection and learning. It is not a simple relationship. Moon (2004a) endeavoured to untangle the relationships and we summarize the account here. The starting point for the exploration of emotion and reflection was the concept of emotional intelligence – which might have seemed to have all of the answers (Goleman, 1995, 1998). However, the concept is very broad and cannot allow us truly to disentangle the relationships. We therefore treat emotional intelligence as the sensitivity needed when working with the emotions of others.

Clearly it is possible for emotion to be the subject matter of journal-writing or reflection. This is illustrated in the extract from Rainer's book above – the writer talks of her emotional state as the subject matter of her writing (as well as experiencing it). A therapist has to learn about emotional states as subject matter in her educational processes. In addition, however, emotion is involved in different ways in the process of learning and the representation of that learning (e.g. in a journal). However, emotion can arise when we are in the process of writing – and being in a particular emotional state can either block or facilitate reflection. There are different relationships between emotion and reflection here. We illustrate this with an example of a person writing in her journal about war and other aspects of human conflict. Emotion could influence the process:

- where relevant emotion is a conscious influence on the nature of the knowledge (e.g. war, as a concept, may be associated with feelings of fear for one person, or excitement for another);
- where relevant emotion has an influence on the process of learning: as part of our internal experience it influences the manner in which we process new material of learning – e.g. in the journal, the learner is considering people's reactions to the threat of conflict, and she brings expectations that fear will be part of their reaction from her previous learning;
- where relevant emotion arises from the process of learning (i.e. it arises not within the external experience, nor directly in the internal experience that we bring to learning, but within the process of flux between the internal and external experience which results in accommodation). An example here is the sense of excitement that might emerge when the journal writer realizes that her ideas about the origins of a particular conflict are making sense or 'coming together' – or when the solution to a problem becomes evident;
- where emotion that is not directly relevant to the learning situation, affects learning (e.g. in accelerated learning (Beard and Wilson, 2002), 'flow' states

(Csikszentmihalyi, 1990; Claxton, 2000), and 'blocks to learning'). Learning seems to be easier or more difficult because of the emotional state – writing in the journal is made more difficult because of the distraction of a new boyfriend – or easier because the journal writer has taken her journal outside on a warm early summer day and feels positive, but particularly introspective.

We have suggested various ways in which emotion plays a part in reflective learning or journal activities. The question is whether this is now the complete list. Consider the following:

- A student teacher writes in her learning journal about a painful incident that occurred when she was at school. It was an incident that has always bothered her. She reads a novel and talks with a friend about how the content relates to her experience and suddenly she sees the incident in a different light. This influences the whole of her orientation to teaching – worries fall away and she feels 'different'.
- The subject in Rainer's diary extract (above) undergoes the catharsis that she anticipates, and her whole outlook feels different.

We have coined the term 'emotional insight' for these changes. The literature on learning and emotion does not seem to have a term for this – and, as the first example demonstrates, it can be very relevant to journal processes. Donaldson, in her book *Human Minds* (1992) uses a schema for the process of learning that could be taken to imply the existence of this process. She uses examples from the literature on spirituality and eastern philosophies (e.g. Bhuddism) to illustrate it, and suggests that the western ways of thinking have not recognized such forms of experience and learning. 'Emotional insight' would seem to be a form of learning that is not a conscious process in that it is not immediately accessible to description in terms of language.

We end this section by bringing it back to the beginning. Journal-writing is a process that enables us to experience, address, explore, manage and work with emotion. Sometimes, too, emotion may 'get in the way' of what is intended in the learning and may seem not to be enhancing conditions favourable for the 'intended' learning – but it may be that other learning ensues. We end, however, on the suggestion that emotion is always present in our learning and journal-writing processes, influencing them in a wide range of ways (Damasio, 2000).

Journals give learners an experience of dealing with ill-structured material of learning

Perhaps one of the most important ways in which journal-writing provides a condition that accentuates conditions under which learning is enhanced is because journal-writing tends to deal with situations that are not 'straightforward'. King and Kitchener (1994) use the phrase 'ill-structured'. They define 'ill-structured' problems as those that 'cannot be described with a high degree of completeness', that 'cannot be resolved with a high degree of certainty' and where experts 'may disagree about the best solution, even when the problem can be considered solved' (1994: 11). Specific examples are the discussion of ethical decisions or the task that Field set for herself in finding out what made her happy (Field, 1952). These are not problems where the educational goal is to find the correct answer, but the goal is to 'construct and defend reasonable solutions' (King and Kitchener, 1994: 11).

King and Kitchener (1994) found that the ability of subjects to cope with ill-structured material is related to their level of epistemological sophistication, their ability to understand that what we know is constructed from what seems to be the most reasonable at the time. It is therefore provisional and subject to re-evaluation, and conclusions about ill-structured issues are drawn with account taken of the best facts available at the time. The understanding is that the knowledge of others is constructed differently and that their well-argued case can have equal validity.

King and Kitchener worked with thousands of subjects over a period of ten years to develop the scale of reflective judgement. The scale is largely based on the development of epistemological sophistication of subjects and their ability to work with ill-structured material. The writers suggest that the capacities of subjects who function at the top end of the scale are similar to those associated with wisdom. They indicate that the ability to progress in reflective judgement depends on educational activities that are provided by work in for example, ill-structured situations such as those found in much journal-writing. They suggest, for example, that students are familiarized with and expected to work with such challenging issues within their disciplines. They should be encouraged to explore different points of view on a topic, to understand that there are different interpretations, to make judgements and to explain their beliefs. Others, who have done similarly relevant work on epistemology are Belenky *et al.* (1986) and Baxter Magolda (1992, 1994, 1996, 1999 and 2001).

The developmental importance of encountering ill-structured material indicates that a problem in the expanding current higher education system might be the provision of more 'ready-made' material to students – handouts, or lecture notes on the Internet (Furendi, 2005). We 'tidy up', thereby, the training ground of material that is ill-structured, challenging and problematic and we remove a very important source of learning. Challenging students' learning in structured learning journals can help to replace this opportunity for important learning. Through encouragement, training or by their inclination, students can be required to write about the issues that are problematic to them or problematic within their learning, and for which a direct answer is not forthcoming. This challenges their uncertainties and acknowledges problems that need to be resolved (Moon, 2005d).

We conclude this section with a comment from a nurse on her personal experience of journal-writing. The comment beautifully captures her learning from the experience of working on ill-structured issues:

all the turning back and turning over and again. I felt I was pushing myself into corners and forcing myself to stay there until I'd worked out a valid response . . . And then it got worse as I took it more seriously. Back in the corners again and this time instead of crawling around muttering, I felt I had to stand up and confront the corners. It did feel like bumping around in the dark. Then it began to dawn on me. I was refusing to see that it was me who had to switch on the lights. And the switches . . . generally . . . were just above my head.

(Ghaye and Lillyman, 1997: 74)

Journals encourage metacognition (learning about one's own process of learning)

We start with a quotation from Jaye (2001). Jaye was interested in her own process of learning and following a holiday, wrote accounts of what she had learnt in the holiday on a number of occasions at increasing distance in time from the holiday – forming thereby a retrospective journal that focused on metacognition. In one entry she was concerned with the process of memory:

Another event made me aware of by the manner in which a journal account of events provides a framework for reconstruction of memory. A number of times during the holiday I wondered what places I had visited in previous visits to Cornwall – most visits had involved touring. While I did not recall what places looked like, I felt that names were very familiar. A week or so after I got back, I located details of the main previous visit in a diary of over 30 years ago. From the scaffolding of the account, I recalled other aspects of that visit. I think if I went back to the same account, I would regain more· memories – but, of course, the notion of 'reconstruction' comes in – are my recollections 'real' or what I am constructing as 'reality'? Does it matter if they are real or what I think are real? I am aware that it may not matter to me personally – but if others were involved, and the event was of significance – that would matter.

(Jaye, 2001)

Metacognition is defined as 'knowledge and cognition about . . . anything cognitive' or 'anything psychological' (Flavell, 1987: 21) and 'the ability to monitor one's current state of learning' (Brown *et al.*, 1986: 66). Sometimes the idea of ability to control one's cognitive strategies is included in the definition (Hadwin and Winne, 1996; Flavell, 1987), though Prawat (1989) prefers to restrict the references to the control aspects of cognition.

Journal-writing has been associated with improved capacities for metacognition directly (McCrindle and Christensen, 1995) or by implication (Boud, 2001; Gillis, 2001), and metacognitive capabilities have been related to an individual's capacity to study effectively or to learn (Hadwin and Winne, 1996; Ertmer and Newby,

1996). It might seem, therefore, that the development of metacognitive abilities may be a further explanation for the support that journal-writing provides for general aspects of learning.

A number of papers discuss the importance of metacognitive knowledge in the learning process. For example, Paris and Winograd say: 'The central message is that students can enhance their learning by becoming aware of their own thinking as they read, write and solve problems . . . A great deal of research supports the importance of metacognition in cognitive development and academic learning' – though they admit to metacognition being a 'fuzzy concept' (1990: 15). It is suggested that the greater ability in learning is achieved by a continuous comparison of the performance of cognitive processes with the goals that the learner is set to reach. The information is used to monitor or guide the learning strategies that are utilized (Weinstein, 1987). However, it also seems likely that greater metacognitive capacities also mean that learners are more aware of, or more able to define, the goals for their learning, themselves.

The role of reflection is suggested to be particularly significant in more sophisticated learning. Ertmer and Newby (1996) see reflection as the 'link' between metacognitive knowledge and self-regulation: 'Reflection makes it possible for learners to utilize their metacognitive knowledge about task, self, and strategies during each stage of the regulatory process: planning, monitoring and evaluating.' The authors see metacognitive knowledge as 'static' and reflection as the more 'active process'. In a reciprocal manner, it will become evident in the next chapter, that the capacity to deliberate about one's own cognitive processes is an important characteristic of the most sophisticated stage of reflective writing (Moon, 2004a).

The theorizing of the paragraph above is reflected in the practical approach of McCrindle and Christensen (1995). These writers link journal-writing, enhanced metacognitive capacity and the enhancement of learning in a discipline. They propose a model of learning in which metacognition and a person's conception of the nature of learning determine the choice of cognitive strategy adopted for the learning task, and these, in turn, affect performance. They tested their model through experimental work with 40 first-year biology students, 20 of whom kept a journal and the other half of whom wrote a scientific report in the same time. Those writing journals were asked to reflect on the nature of their learning in the laboratory classes and there was an opportunity, therefore, for the journals to influence their metacognitive awareness. The results indicated that the journal writers generally performed better than the report group in the class examination. Their knowledge was of better quality and better structured. They used more advanced strategies for learning and had greater metacognitive awareness about their tasks. In terms of their conceptions of learning, there was a considerable difference between the two groups, the journal writers viewing learning in a more sophisticated manner. As a result of this work, McCrindle and Christensen conclude, 'The provision of opportunities to deliberately reflect on their own learning can constitute a significant instructional innovation for tertiary students.'

It would be interesting to know, in this research, how the journal-writing in biology affected learning in other subject areas.

We end this section on a cautionary note which is introduced at the end of the quotation from Jaye (2001). How do we know that what we report in journal or other writing as our cognitive processes are indeed the real processes that we underwent – and not a reconstruction of them? An old paper by Nisbett and DeCamp Wilson (1977) discusses experimental work on this issue and throws doubts on the ease of access and accuracy of reporting of subjects on their own processes – but maybe reconstruction is helpful too . . .

Journals enhance learning through the process of writing

Writing is a form of representation of learning, a means of demonstrating what we have learnt and importantly, a tool for the enhancement of more learning (Moon, 2005a, 2005c). While it may be relatively easy for teachers to accept the learning role of writing when they apply it to their own activities such as drafting and redrafting a paper, in class, many only utilize writing as a means of expression or communication. In this mode, it is the manner in which words convey meaning and factors such as their grammatical correctness that raise comment, not the learning that might have accrued for the student in the process. In some disciplines, such as mathematics, writing may hardly be used at all and this represents a lost opportunity. Even in subjects like this, writing can be used effectively to promote learning as Chapter 6 demonstrates (Selfe *et al.*, 1986).

The value of writing as an important means of learning has been discussed by a series of writers whose work is often quoted in support of the use of learning journals in education. Richardson puts these different viewpoints in context: 'I write because I want to find something out. I write in order to learn something I didn't know before I wrote it' (Richardson, 1994: 517).

Formal writing as it occurs in formal educational settings is normally not the same as the form in which personal journals are written. In encouraging students to write journals, we are usually asking them to write in a form that few would have used in formal educational contexts. The relatively informal language – termed 'expressive language', described by Parker and Goodkin as 'comfortable, ready to hand language' (1987: 14) – is to be used in situations 'which are new, puzzling, troubling or intriguing' (1987: 14), and when we are exploring and thinking through writing 'in which a writer gets into a relationship' with an issue.

Relatively few of those concerned with journal-writing note the significance of the different forms of language used in many journals and other educational tasks. However, some do. Weil (1996) notes the value of first-person writing even at the level of the doctorate. Selfe *et al.* (1986) worked with mathematics students who were asked in their journals to write, in their own language, about mathematical concepts. Among other findings, the writers note that: 'The act of writing . . . in

their own language and using their own experience helped students seal ...
concepts and problems in their mind' (1986: 201).

The term 'expressive writing' was used by Britton (1972). Britton based the
theory of his writing on Bruner's (1971) work on language and thought. In an often-
cited paper, Emig (1977) also related the use of writing for learning to Bruner's
work. She referred to Bruner's suggestion that we learn in three different ways –
though doing (enactive), though imagery (iconic) and through representational or
symbolic means. 'What is striking about writing as a process', she says, 'is that, by
its very nature, all three ways of dealing with actuality are simultaneously, or almost
simultaneously deployed.' She suggests that in this way, writing 'through its
inherent reinforcing cycle involving hand, eye and brain marks a uniquely powerful multi-representational mode for learning'. In addition Emig argues that the
involvement of both brain hemispheres implies that 'writing involves the fullest
functioning of the brain'.

We summarize some of the means by which learning from writing occurs.
Clearly some of these points relate back to other headings in this chapter – there
is reciprocity and there are multiple dimensions – and this is one of the values of
the journal as a learning tool.

- Writing forces time to be taken for reflection (Holly and McLoughlin, 1989).
- Writing forces learners to organize and to clarify their thoughts in order to
  sequence in a linear manner. In this way they reflect on and improve their
  understanding (Moon, 1999b).
- Writing causes learners to focus their attention. It forces activity in the learner.
- Writing helps learners to know whether or not they understand something. If
  they cannot explain it, they probably cannot understand it.
- Along similar lines, being asked to write the explanation of something
  can encourage a deep approach to learning in the manner that the learner
  anticipates the quality of understanding required for the writing (Moon,
  1999b).
- Writing an account of something enables the writer to talk about it more
  clearly (Selfe et al., 1986).
- Writing captures ideas for later consideration.
- Writing sets up a 'self-provided feedback system' (Yinger, 1985).
- Writing can record a train of thought and relate it in past, present and future
  (Emig, 1977).
- The process of writing is creative, and develops new structures. It can be
  enjoyable.
- The pace of writing slows the pace of thinking and can thereby increase its
  effectiveness (Emig, 1977).

There are other qualities in self-expressive writing of the kind that might be found
in journals. These qualities may have a power that sometimes goes beyond
individual words. Elbow says:

I like to call this power 'juice'. The metaphor comes to me again and again. I suppose because I am trying to get at something mysterious and hard to define. 'Juice' combines the qualities of magic potion, mother's milk and electricity. Sometimes I fear I will never be clear about what I mean by voice . . . in writing. [It] implies words that capture the sound of an individual on the page . . . Writing with no voice is dead, mechanical, faceless. It lacks any sound.

(Elbow, 1981: 286–7)

Thinkpoint

There was a garden shed in my father's small garden where I kept rabbits and a tame raven. There I spent endless hours, long as geological ages in warmth and blissful ownership; the rabbits smelled of life, of grass and milk, of blood and procreation; and in the raven's hard, black eye shone the lamp of eternal life. In the same place I spent other endless epochs in the evenings, beside a guttering candle with the warm, sleeping animals . . . and sketched out plans for discovering immense treasures, finding the mandrake root and launching victorious crusades on which I would execute robbers, free miserable captives, raze thieves strongholds . . . forgive runaway vassals, win king's daughters and understand the language of animals.

(Hesse, 1975: 25)

To express these thoughts or attitudes towards life seemed to me only possible by means of fairy tales.

(Hesse, 1975: 65)

Chapter 4

Quality and depth in reflection and learning journals

This chapter will provide a brief introduction to some definitions of reflection and reflective learning and then consider how these relate to the way in which learners write reflectively in learning journals. Some considerations that underpin this chapter relate to the experiences of teachers who choose to use journals with their students: that some students have difficulty in starting with reflective writing and that when they do get started and can write in a reflective 'kind of' way, the nature of the reflective writing of most learners is superficial and descriptive and probably does not lead to deep or comprehensive learning (Lyons, 1999; Samuals and Betts, 2005). Development work has been done on this issue since the first edition of this book and this chapter details the new ideas. Some of this chapter is close to material in Moon (2004a).

Definitions of reflection and reflective learning

Moon (1999a) set out to clarify the nature of reflection having observed the complexity of the literature in this area. Some of the literature, for example, seems to suggest that reflection is no more than a form of thinking (the 'commonsense view of reflection' – see below). However this kind of view does not accord with the manner in which reflection is often operationalized in formal education (the academic view of reflection – see below). Complicating the situation, too, is the literature from various disciplines, including education, professional development and psychology, that appears to use the idea of reflection in many different ways.

The commonsense view of reflection

A commonsense view of reflection is developed by examination of how we use the word 'reflection' in everyday language. We have said that reflection is akin to thinking – but there is more to be added to this. We may reflect in order to achieve an outcome, or for some purpose or we may simply 'be reflective', and an outcome might then be unexpected. Reflection is an activity that we apply to more complex issues. We do not reflect on the route to the bus-stop, or on how to do a simple arithmetical sum where there is an obvious solution. We think it through or plan it. However, we might reflect on whether or not to complain about something when this action may generate difficult consequences. In addition the content of reflection is, as we have suggested in Chapter 2, largely what we know already. It is often a process of re-organizing knowledge and emotional orientations in order to achieve further insights – we used the term 'cognitive housekeeping' to imply the sense of reordering what is there already.

On the basis of the reasoning above, a commonsense view of reflection can be stated as follows:

> Reflection is a form of mental processing – like a form of thinking – that we may use to fulfil a purpose or to achieve some anticipated outcome or we may simply 'be reflective' and then an outcome can be unexpected. Reflection is applied to relatively complicated, ill-structured ideas for which there is not an obvious solution and is largely based on the further processing of knowledge and understanding that we already possess.

Reflection applied in academic contexts: a development of the commonsense view – and some myths

Since the late 1990s, the theory and practice of reflection has attained a much more significant role in educational contexts. Unless there is clarity about the strictures that tend to be imposed upon reflection in these specific contexts, there is a danger that we make the technical an everyday activity. Reflection that is a requirement of a curriculum is likely to have some characteristics that are specified in advance. On this basis, it is useful to add a different kind of view of reflection in order to encompass its application in the academic context. It would not be appropriate in academia, for example, to say that professional development is enhanced when a person goes for a sunny walk in a reflective mood. We would require something more tangible and directed – or the reflection might be expected to occur within a given structure. An element of the structure is likely to be a description of an incident. Furthermore, the outcome of reflection, which is most likely to be reflective writing, is usually seen by a tutor, and is often assessed. This can lead to some students writing the 'reflective' material that they think will be viewed favourably by their tutor (Salisbury, 1994). In addition, evidence of learning or change of behaviour may be expected to result from the process of reflection. These factors are also likely to influence the nature of reflective learning (Boud and Walker, 1998).

On the basis of the paragraph above, we add to the commonsense definition of reflection as follows:

> Reflection/reflective learning or reflective writing in the academic context is also likely to involve a conscious and stated purpose for the reflection, with

an outcome specified in terms of learning, action or clarification. It may be preceded by a description of the purpose and/or the subject matter of the reflection. The process and outcome of reflective work is most likely to be in a represented (e.g. written) form, to be seen by others and to be assessed. All of these factors can influence its nature and quality.

In practice, the way in which reflection is used in educational situations is often quite narrowly defined. For example it may be defined in terms of learning from recognized error or ineffectiveness in practice (Hinett, 2003; Mackintosh, 1998). In addition it is often subject to a set of beliefs – which might actually be called 'myths'. These views are worth considering here since they can obstruct further understanding. The three 'myths' are that

- 'emotion is central to reflective processes'
- 'reflection is about "my own" processes' (i.e. always in the first person)
- 'some people cannot reflect'.

We have discussed the various roles of emotion in learning. Some people consider that reflection is actually characterized by its emotional components. Some suggestions are: that reflection and feeling act in interdependent relationship with emotion (Taylor, 1997); that emotion is represented sometimes as tacit knowledge (McAlpine and Weston, 2002); that past emotional experience 'highlights' issues to be dealt with (Mezirow, 1998; Boud and Walker, 1998); or that reflective learning may demand 'emotional stamina' (Mezirow, 1998). In Chapter 3 we made an assumption that emotion is intimately involved in all learning – not just reflection. A number of different relationships between emotion and learning were identified and we suggest that any of these can be operative in reflection. It is possible that the nature of reflective activity leads to greater awareness of emotion and greater account being taken of the role of emotion but we would not say that emotional involvement characterizes reflection. Some possibilities are that:

- there may be a more permissive attitude towards the involvement of emotion in reflective activity than in other areas of formal education;
- since reflection involves the 'slowing of the pace of learning' (see below), it is easier to recognize the role of emotion in the process of learning when it is slowed down;
- journals tap emotional insight (Chapter 3) and this form of learning is not common in other academic work;
- reflective learning encourages metacognitive consideration of the role of emotion in learning.

It may be that all of these are relevant.

Another myth is that reflection always concerns the self – in other words, it is always about the role of the 'first person' (I . . .). From asking participants at workshops what they think reflective learning 'is about', it would seem that this is a common conception. There seems to be no reason why this should be the case, although the self does tend to be central in many of the ways in which reflection is applied in formal educational contexts, for example in professional development and in personal appraisal. It is perfectly possible, though, to reflect on factors that are not personal – for example, on morality issues in a relationship whether it is one's own relationship, or that of others, or on how students responded to a particular idea.

Lastly there is the myth that some people cannot reflect. We have said – and it is the subject of further consideration later – that when asked to reflect in formal educational situations, many learners resist or have difficulty in understanding what they should do (Boud and Walker, 1998; Jasper, 1998; Tomlinson, 1999; Lucas, 2001). In contrast, other learners will have no difficulty and will not understand the problems encountered by their colleagues. There are cultural norms that may lead to a resistance to 'navel-gazing'. Since reflection is suggested to be an element in good quality forms of learning, we take the position that everyone can reflect, though this may not always be a conscious activity and may not be done willingly when required. The acceptability of overt reflective processes may be related to different practices in disciplines. Assuming that everyone can reflect does not mean that everyone uses reflection effectively to improve her performance. Ferry and Ross-Gordon (1998) and McAlpine and Weston (2002) present evidence that professionals vary in the effectiveness with which they utilize reflection and that this is not just a function of their level of experience. It is also possible that while everyone can reflect, some do have genuine difficulty with representing their reflection in writing. There may be some gender differences here.

Reflection: its quality and depth

We introduced this chapter by the suggestion that it can be difficult to persuade learners (particularly in an academic context) to represent their more than superficially. This was a uneasy observation that remained unresolved in the writing of the first edition of this book.

We use the terminology 'levels of reflection' to imply a hierarchical model of reflective activity that demonstrates progression from what is little different from description, to a profound form of reflection. Most models that incorporate the notion of depth of reflection do not imply that the levels are qualitatively different, though they may use specific terms for the different levels (e.g. Van Manen, 1977). In the model that is developed in this book, qualitative differences between the levels are acknowledged.

Some examples of work on the depth quality of reflection are Hettich (1976, 1990); Van Manen (1977); Wedman and Martin (1986); Ross (1989); Sparkes-Langer et al. (1990); Sparkes-Langer and Colton (1991); Hatton and Smith Kember et al. (1999) and Kember et al. (2000). Generally this material seems to be consistent, attributing similar qualities to the deeper levels of reflection and generally viewing superficial reflection as descriptive. However, little of the work seems to have been taken into general use in the classroom, possibly because it has been too theoretical for direct use by learners.

In the frameworks described in the references above, deep reflection is generally characterized by perspective transformation (Mezirow, 1998), or transformative learning (Moon, 1999a). These terms refer to the ability to revise the 'meaning structures' (Taylor, 1997) which are the bases of judgements. In other words, we are talking of the learner reviewing the manner of the functioning of internal experience, what frames of reference are used, and how they are used. In turn this implies a functional understanding of the constructed nature of knowledge and a metacognitive stance. Another quality of deep reflection is its critical orientation to one's own and others' understandings. A number of writers have commented on the inadequacy of much activity performed in the name of reflection because it is non-critical and non-reflective – or non-reflexive (Kim, 1999). Taylor and White (2000) provide a well-illustrated argument of the inadequacy of the reflective practice model and the importance of criticality in professional situations:

> The primary focus of reflection is on process issues ... Its focus on knowledge is primarily confined to the application of 'theory to practice' ... Reflexivity takes things further. Specifically, it problematizes issues that reflection takes for granted ... For example, it assumes that through reflection the worker can become more adept at applying child development and attachment theories more effectively. Reflexivity suggests that we interrogate these previously taken-for-granted assumptions.
>
> (Taylor and White, 2000: 198)

All of those who discern levels of reflection seem to agree with the statement above, but use different terminologies – so 'reflexivity', like 'critical reflection' or perspective transformation would be seen as associated with the deepest level of reflection. In addition, among the theorists there is an implication that deeper reflection yields better quality outcomes in terms of learning.

The work of Hatton and Smith (1995) is probably the best known framework of levels of reflection. This was developed in experimental work on the reflective writing of teacher education students. It was then formulated into a tool for wider use. A brief description of the levels follows (using some of Hatton and Smith's own words):

Descriptive writing Writing that is not considered to show evidence of reflection: it is a description with no discussion beyond description.

Descriptive reflection There is description of events. The possibility of alternative view-points is accepted but most reflection is from one perspective.

Dialogic reflection The work demonstrates 'a "stepping back" from events and actions leading to a different level of mulling about discourse with self and exploring the discourse of events and actions'. There is a recognition that different qualities of judgement and alternative explanations may exist for the same material. The reflection is analytical or integrative, though may reveal inconsistency.

Critical reflection   'Demonstrates an awareness that actions and events are not only located within and explicable by multiple perspectives, but are located in and influenced by multiple historical and socio-political contexts.'
(Quotations from Hatton and Smith, 1995)

Hatton and Smith's work was used with several cohorts of higher education work experience placement learners. For assessment purposes, these students were required to produce a reflective account. Initially the accounts had been disappointing since they were so superficial. The tool therefore had a purpose both for guiding the work of the learners, as well as providing a rationale for assessment purposes (i.e. by providing assessment criteria). An interesting point that became evident in the process of this work is that we should take care not to reject all descriptive writing. Some description is necessary in a reflective account that is used in a formal situation to provide the background for the reflection. However, this 'statement of how things are' has a different role when one is writing from the role of reflection and should not be confused with the latter.

The development of exercises to encourage the deepening of reflection

Despite the apparent value of Hatton and Smith's framework, which the writer began to use in workshops and with students, it was still difficult to help learners properly to understand the nature of deeper reflection. They seemed to need more detail and examples of reflective work in order to understand what was required. A further stage was then to develop an exercise where different levels of reflection are based on one initial descriptive account of a particular situation. The first of these exercises was developed prior to a development session for staff who were being required to be able to write reflectively in order to enter the Institute for Learning and Teaching (ILT). It consisted of a short descriptive story about an incident in a park and two further accounts of the same event that were written at two deeper levels of reflection. The concept of level of reflection was based on the work with Hatton and Smith's model and that of the others mentioned above. Alongside the exercise, a rationale was written for each scenario – indicating the reflective characteristics of it. Subsequently a fourth senario was developed. The resulting exercise has been used widely with staff and students working in small groups. The scenarios are read in sequence, with the group asked to discuss 'how reflective is this' for around five to ten minutes per scenario. When they have processed all of the scenarios in turn, they are asked to note the characteristics of the accounts that have changed from the first to the fourth. This discussion occurs in a plenary session and then the participants are directed towards the rationale. The management of this and others is described in Resource 1 (pp. 159–60). 'The Park' and other exercises like it are provided in Resources 3, 4 and 5 (pp. 164–81). (The resources section can be freely photocopied.)

A few exercises such as those described above were generated, each with its own rationale but later a 'Generic Framework for Reflective Writing' was developed and this has guided the writing of subsequent such exercises (Resource 2, pp. 161–3). Around 2,500 participants (mainly teaching staff, but some students) in workshops in the UK and abroad have now done the exercises. Later we make further reference to this form of exercise in the context of how to start with learning journals (Chapter 9).

The development of the scenario approach to depth in reflective writing has meant that a theoretical issue in reflection (depth and quality) has been tackled through a practical means – and indeed, the writer has learnt much about depth issues in the development and use of the material in workshops. We could say, in the terminology of Fazey and Marton (2002), that increasing depth in reflection relies on an increasing awareness, use of and sophistication in the use of variation in the internal experience (i.e. in cognitive housekeeping processes). Further underpinning theory to the framework is presented in Moon (2004a).

We have suggested that the framework can support teaching staff and students in learning to works with reflective writing and we have suggested that it is a theoretical tool to promote the understanding of what we mean by reflective work – however it is also of value in the process of assessment of reflective work – in that it implies a set of assessment criteria for reflective writing where the quality of the writing is to be assessed (see Chapter 10).

Depth of reflection: some issues to consider

Logically there is no 'end-point' of deep reflection – the journal work could go on and on examining issues in a wider and wider context and at different points of time from the event (if the reflection is on an event) to infinity. However, in most situations in which reflection is applied there will be logistical reasons for limiting the processes of reflection – for example, word limits in the journal in an academic context. An element of strategy is required in most academic reflective writing, therefore, in order to be able to meet given constraints. It has become evident both in the development of the exercises on levels of reflection (see above) and from working with learners, that deeper reflection often requires more word-length than superficial reflection, especially if, within the word length there is to be a short description of the event/issue. It is not unusual to require 'reflective pieces' in journals to be written in (for example) 200 or 500 words. It is the experience of the writer that such tight word limits can inhibit deeper reflection because there is more to write about in deeper reflection. Extending the word limit in some situations has been observed to encourage deeper reflection.

It is also useful to think about the appropriate depth of writing that is required. In the application of staff to join the Institute for Teaching and Learning, it is not necessary that staff should write deep details about their personal attributes as teachers. A reflective, but reasonably superficial account was required. The depth required of student writing is a matter for discussion.

Thinkpoint

This piece was written at Corbridge, Northumberland in July. It is an extract from a written and sketched diary of a exploration of Britain (Bell, 1981: 177). A sketch of woodland accompanies it.

> Spagnum peat and sand dunes are all very well, but when it comes to getting your boots muddy you can't beat the dark earth. This patch of woodland breathes earthiness of an evening. I enjoyed the spectacular scenes of Scotland but there is more than enough to keep me occupied, watching and drawing along this field edge. For me this is almost home territory, an 'ordinary' sort of place. Yet no place is all that ordinary; there is a Roman road a couple of fields away and according to the geological map of Northern Britain, the wood lies close to a geological boundary, a tongue of millstone grit outcrops on this hillside over rocks of the Carboniferous limestone series.

Chapter 5

The uses of learning journals

Introduction

The chapter covers two different aspects of the management of learning journals that have a place somewhere between how we learn from journals (Chapters 2, 3 and 4), and their more practical place in education, professions and living (Chapters 6, 7, 8 and 9).

The first section of this chapter interprets the word 'use' in terms of values or purposes. In previous work we have indicated that there are a large number of purposes for journal-writing that are cited in the literature (Moon, 1999a). These purposes are not always identified by those who initiate journal work. It is often the case that learners are simply asked to write journals with no purpose being formally specified. Making the purpose as clear as possible for learners is of crucial importance for helping learners to start to write, and in the relationship which that purpose should have to bear on any assessment or feedback processes (Fenwick, 2001). Where purpose has not been specified, at the stage of assessment or evaluation there are often indications that a purpose lurked there which (unfairly on learners) was not voiced.

The purposes of journals

We list some purposes for using learning journals below. Most journal-writing would serve several of the following purposes whether or not the purposes are made explicit, and some of the purposes subsume others. Those purposes which are covered in greater detail in other chapters in this book, are merely sketched out here. The following is a list of purposes for journal-writing and it represents a revised version of those in Moon (1999a).

To record experience

For perhaps most of those who write journals, the primary purpose may be to 'record experience', but then also to process it further (Brockbank and McGill, 1998). For some, the emphasis may be on the recording (Wolf, 1980) which may be akin to the development of a log in its objectivity. Such recording may, for example, parallel research, professional or project activity (Holly, 1989; Brookfield, 1995; Stephani, 1997; Glaze, 2002; Talbot, 2002). In many current initiatives, experience is recorded in the past or present and accompanied by a reflective record that can take the form of reflective writing or journal activities. These may be in the form of portfolios (Burke and Rainbow, 1998) or profiles (James, 1993), records of achievement/experience (James and Denley, 1993), progress files (NCIHE, 1997), or in personal development profiles/plans (Cottrell, 2003) – see Chapter 6. Some other examples of the use of journals where the emphasis is on recording experience include the use of journals to record experience in clinical (dental) situations which is beyond the requirements of the curriculum (Oliver, 1998). Another is the use of a log by clients in psychotherapy sessions (Fox, 1982) and in another example, students used journals to record their discussions with 'live' teenagers in a psychology of adolescence course (McManus, 1986).

To facilitate learning from experience

While some journals are primarily for the recording of experience, others emphasize the processes of reflection that follow the experience. This is the case for many of the journals in professional education and development, particularly those that follow either the Kolb cycle of experiential learning (Kolb, 1984) or the work of Schön on reflection-on-action (Schön, 1983). Parker and Goodkin describe the role of language in first 'interpreting our interpretations' (1987: 176).

On a broader basis, journals that accompany field work or work experience provide a method of developing the meaning of experiences so that learners can relate their unique experience to established theory, or to develop their own theory. Walker (1985) describes the use of a portfolio to support learning on a course for those who would be leaders of religious communities. All of the teaching staff encouraged the use of the portfolio, the aim of which was to record learning experiences in order to reflect on their implications for personal development. There are many other examples of journals where the purpose is to learn from experience: Orem, 2001; Gillis, 2001; Shepherd, 2004. Moon (2004a) links reflective learning to experiential learning and learning from experience.

To support understanding and the representation of the understanding

The use of journals to support learning is generally applied in most uses of journal-writing and the role of learning in journal-writing is explored in Chapter 2. Some examples in which the role of journals in learning is specified as a purpose are Wetherell and Mullins (1996), who used journals on a problem-based learning programme to ensure the integration of learning, and Meese (1987) and Parker and

Goodkin (1987) who have used journals to 'focus' learning. Ficher (1990) used journals to facilitate and clarify thinking and Wagenaar (1984), Hettich (1976) and Terry (1984) used journals in different academic programmes to enhance academic learning by linking it with everyday experiences of their disciplines. This might well improve learning through improvement of motivation and the encouragement of a deep approach to learning (Mortimer, 1998). Others have talked about the way that journals are a means of slowing down learning, ensuring that learners take more thorough account of situations. They change the pace of learning (e.g. Jensen, 1987). Christensen (1981) considers that journal-writing is a means of safeguarding learners against the push towards expectations of greater volumes of learning to be achieved more and more quickly. Stephani, Clarke and Littlejohn (2000) used 'logbooks' to enable the students in higher education to feel more involved with the expectations and structure of their programme.

To develop critical thinking or the development of a questioning attitude

It is also common to associate journal-writing with the improvement of thinking skills (Moon, 2005d). This category of purpose, however, is also associated with critical thinking and questioning towards social change. Smyth (1989), in particular, focuses on the raising of social and professional consciousness as a purpose for journal-writing. Other relevant examples of journal or reflective writing are Tsang (2003), Ledwith (2005), and Trelfa (2005). Moon suggests the use of journals as a means of enhancing the development of critical thinking and epistemological maturity.

To encourage metacognition

Chapter 2 mentions a number of writers who are interested in the enhancement of metacognitive capacities as an experimental outcome of journal-writing. Others imply an expectation that learners will become more aware of their learning processes. For example, Mülhaus and Löschmann (1997) sought to improve the learning strategies of their students of German by asking them to take note of their learning in journals. Hettich (1990) introduced psychology students to models of thinking, and considered that with careful introduction, the parallel use of this material with journal-writing could enhance student thinking. There can be a greater justification for knowledge of personal learning in situations in the education of educators, for example Morrison (1996), working in teacher education. Handley (1998), working with IT trainers, used journals to generate understanding of the limitations of personal learning styles that might be presumed to affect their training styles. Another valuable example of metacognition in a journal is that of Glaze (2002), who provides a reflective commentary on her use of a journal during the period of her PhD 'so that the PhD experience could be brought to life'.

To increase active involvement in and ownership of learning

Developing a sense of ownership of material is a condition that facilitates learning (Chapter 3). Writing a journal can have the effect of bringing knowledge presented as 'out there' into the ownership of the writer. It involves working with meanings and ensuring that the meanings relate to the current understanding of the writer. 'It thrusts the student into an active role in the classroom' (Jensen, 1987: 333). Tama and Peterson (1991) demonstrate this engagement in their use of literature to encourage reflection in student teachers. Shepherd's comment about the journal that he used when working as a volunteer management advisor in Cambodia provides insight into his sense of ownership of his journal and the learning that it supported. He says 'I started to value my journal . . . for the power it had to bring about change in me . . . (It) took on a preciousness I associate with artifacts of personal value, like that of an old photograph album' (Shepherd, 2004).

To increase ability in reflection and thinking

Journal-writing and reflection are linked in Chapter 2, both in general terms and in the manner in which we have suggested that reflection is fundamental to the taking of a deep approach to learning (Moon, 1999a, 2004a; Stephani, 1997).

To enhance problem-solving skills

In some of the areas of the curriculum in which journal-writing might seem less likely – in the sciences, applied sciences and quantitative disciplines – the value of writing has been demonstrated in the process of problem solving (Jensen, 1987; Grumbacher, 1987; Korthagan, 1988; Cowan, 1998a). More is said of this in Chapter 6.

As a means of assessment in formal education

While we will argue in Chapter 10 that there are advantages and difficulties associated with the assessment of journals, there is no reason why journal-writing should not be set explicitly for the purpose of assessment. The result may be a less free-thinking version of a journal, although that depends on the nature of the assessment criteria which are set in advance or which the learners perceive to govern their attainment of grades.

One example of journals as an assessment form is Burnard (1988), working with student nurses. In the context of education for returning adults, Redwine (1989) describes a reflective account that accompanied a submission for the assessment of prior experiential learning. This, in turn, would give exemption from parts of a programme of learning. In a more focused example, Fazey describes how she introduced student self-assessment diaries into the process of personal skill development (Fazey, 1993). Similarly, seeing assessment as a means of monitoring progress, Wetherell and Mullins (nd) provide an example in dentistry.

To enhance reflective practice

As Chapter 7 will indicate, professional practice is a broad area of activity that probably includes most of the purposes of journal use that are listed in this chapter. On this basis it is interesting to note that it is in the professional development literature that the predominance of literature on journals lies. A particular reason for using journals in professional education is to enhance reflective practice. Reflective practice seems to come in many guises and is therefore difficult to 'pin down'. Betts (2004) discusses the concept and concludes that it is far more contentious than would be evident from the manner in which the term is used. Her experiences involved the use of journals with management students.

For reasons of personal development and self-empowerment

The use of journals to enhance and develop the self is the subject matter of Chapter 8. As a topic it overlaps in particular with professional development. Some would say that professional development inevitably involves personal development (Harvey and Knight, 1996). It is also the case that many of the purposes listed here could contribute to the empower–mentor development of the self. On another view, the nature of journal-writing means that there is an exploration of self and the personal meanings and constructs through which one views the world that is implicit in most effective journal-writing (Christensen, 1981; Walker, 1985; Grumet, 1990; Morrison, 1996; Moon, 1999a; Shepherd, 2004). An interesting view of the notion of empowerment in association with learning journals is described in Stockhausen and Kawashima (2002), who used journals with a group of Japanese nurses. A revealing quotation from one of the nurses who was interviewed in the research was:

> As the workbook proceeded, I found that the questions asked were expanded to a variety of nursing issues such as the position of nurses in the health care system, society and their status, etc. When I considered these significant contexts, I started to be excited and wanted to know more about how I could use reflective practice to extend myself professionally.
>
> (Stockhausen and Kawashima, 2002)

However, there are some uses of journals that are directed specifically towards the use of journals to explore the personal world, such as that of Progoff (1975) and those who followed him. There is also a group, like Field, who set out to find out about aspects of personal behaviour to bring it under better personal control (Field, 1952; Rainer, 1978).

For therapeutic purposes or as a means of supporting behaviour change

One origin of Progoff's work towards development of the Intensive Journal was in the context of psychotherapy sessions where he suggested that patients should keep a note of the 'events of their inner life' as they emerged during and between the therapy sessions. This appeared to have a valuable therapeutic effect and he extended it by 'drawing forward the inner processes' through questions and discussion (Progoff, 1975: 26–7). Fox (1982) used a similar technique with good results.

Used in the personal context, a journal can act as a place symbolically to offload the burden of unpleasant events or experiences, an 'emotional dumping ground' (Moon, 1999b). It can act as a way of working through difficult feelings, perhaps by writing letters that are not actually sent or for clarifying conflicts and working out guilt (Cooper, 1991). It was noted earlier that a number of successful writers seem to have worked through deprivations in the earlier parts of their lives through journals or other personal writing (Storr, 1988).

Reflection in journals can note or log behaviours that are irritating for the individual or for others and reduce their frequency or 'grip'. For example, a journal can be helpful for the maintenance of a diet or other such behaviour change routine.

To enhance creativity

A number of writers talk about the relationship of journal-writing and creativity. Journals may be used to generate creative ideas either at random or through focus on a particular project, or they can record and facilitate the development of the project itself. An example of a journal that facilitated the initiation and subsequent writing of this book is included in Chapter 11. In addition, there is broad use of learning journals in work with art and design students, where the journal may be partially graphic and might coincide with the artist's 'notebook'.

There are a number of suggestions as to how creativity is generated through journal-writing. Milner's (1957) work on learning to draw suggests that one way is by taking account of the unconscious. Miller (1979) says that, as we write conscious thoughts, 'useful associations and new ideas begin to emerge', and writing the immediate thoughts 'makes more "room" for new avenues of thinking'. Through slowing down and taking better account of the 'inner movement of our lives', Christensen (1981) suggests that intuitive elements of the self can 'break through' and give rise to creative insight. In contrast to these, Schneider and Killick (1998) and Mansfield and Bidwell (2005) approach the same subject matter from the angle of creative writing. They suggest that by using journals and self-discovery exercises, readers can find ease in writing from personal experience and thereby may improve their creative writing skills. This kind of approach is linked to the expanding area of work on the use of personal story in self and professional development (see Chapter 11).

To improve writing

The improvement of writing is one of the more common explicit purposes for journal-writing in formal situations (e.g. Brodsky and Meagher, 1987). There are a number of reports on the improvement of writing that has followed the use of journals. For example, Jensen (1987) noted that physics students who wrote journals displayed improved fluency in their essays writing. However, in journal-writing, 'fluency can . . . become gush'. Berthoff (1987: 14) points out the importance of maintaining fluency within the bounds of a structure which makes it productive. The improvement of writing ability may sometimes result from the opportunity that journal-writing provides for integrating everyday language into more academic forms (Parker and Goodkin, 1987; Macrorie, 1970).

To improve or give 'voice'; as a means of self-expression

Some learners are not as able as others at self-expression. Journals provide a means of enabling them to express themselves in an alternative manner (Bowman, 1983). There are different ways of learning and of expressing that learning. Some have much to express, but are not in suitable social or emotionally suitable situations for that expression. Journal-writing is an alternative voice. Craig contrasts finding a voice of one's own with finding a voice 'that we think is proper to share with other people' and notes that it is then that 'we often lose our own voice' (Dillon, 1983). Along similar lines, Peterson and Jones say: 'Women's journals provide a glimpse into the lives of women and into a history that had no space for women's voices. Journals have helped to raise the consciousness of those women who believed the myths that led to their own self-degradation' (Peterson and Jones, 2001: 59).

To foster communication and to foster reflective and creative interaction in a group

Many talk about the use of interaction as a means of facilitating journal-writing for individuals and there is literature on dialogue journals which are shared by two or more people (see later). However, some writers have mentioned a purpose of journal-writing to be to facilitate interaction within a group (Walker, 1985) and Hickman describes the development at what might be the extremes of journal-writing – the office log to 'maintain communication and continuity' (1987: 391). In a number of evaluations of the use of journals in classroom situations for other purposes, there are incidental comments to the effect that students seem more willing to interact in class as a result of their writing.

To support planning and progress in research or a project

Journals may be concerned with quite specific issues – such as the work in one discipline in formal education. They may focus on one piece of work in which the writer is engaged at the time or is planning – such as a research project, a forthcoming event or trip (Holly, 1989). In this context, they become a repository of ideas, plans and thoughts that can greatly enhance the final product or the specific planning of the product. Perhaps the significant difference that the use of a journal during planning makes is that it encourages the practitioner to see planning as a process that occurs over a period of time instead of on one occasion. Ideas can be put down and modified or abandoned – the material is generally mulled over for a while and given time to settle into its most promising format.

There are a number of examples of journals that support specific work such as projects or short courses in Chapter 11. Glaze (2002) and Shepherd (2004) provide further examples.

As a means of communication between a learner and another

A general comment in a number of papers is that a sometimes unexpected outcome of asking students to write journals is that staff learn much more about their students as people and as learners (e.g. Wetherell and Mullins, 1996). The staff learn also about the students' perception of the course itself. In some situations a major purpose of the journal is to maintain the contact between a tutor or mentor and a student who may be in a location at some distance. An example of a use like this is where teaching students are involved in teaching practice in schools at some distance from the university. Email instead of pen and paper is used in this situation for communication (for example, weekly 'chunks' of journal are transmitted from student to tutor who then has an opportunity to comment on the material and transmit the comment back to the student (Parnell, 1998)).

A more equalized way of using dialogue between tutor and student is the dialogue journal format which is described below.

Forms of journal-writing

Journals come in any shape, size or form. They exist as the five-year diary with prescribed space for each day, they could exist as yellow sticky notes stuck on the walls of a room, or they exist not on paper at all. They may be in electronic form on audio or videotape or in a word-processed format and, no doubt, they have been written on stone or the walls of caves. The possibilities are as broad as the imagination of the writer – or of the person who has set journal-writing as a task. However, a more significant factor for the learning result of journal-writing is the internal structure of a journal. Writing, for example, might result from the stimulus of an exercise or a question posed, rather than only existing in the free-flowing form which is initiated directly by the writer. We explore here some of the more usual formats of journals and why particular formats might be chosen. There are four major divisions in this discussion. They represent the relatively unstructured journal, and those that are structured in some way and are written by individuals, and dialogue and other forms of journals that are, in effect, written conversation between two or more people. The fourth form that we discuss here is personal development plans/profiles (PDP) that are often in the form of what could be called journal and are widely used in the UK (see later in this chapter).

The difference between all four forms of journal is somewhat arbitrary. Some entries of individual journals are shared sometimes or seen by a tutor – and structured and unstructured forms of journal are more on a continuum than two separate categories. It is often good practice to start with a journal that is relatively structured and move on to a freer format. Sometimes a structure is provided as an option that the writers may discard if they do not need the support that structure provides. PDP formats are often in the form of highly structured (and often highly regulated) journals.

It may surprise some that we do not make the distinction between electronic and paper-based journals. At the time of writing this second edition of this book, there are many more electronic journal forms in use (in particular in the context of personal development planning). However, this book concerns the principles behind working on a learning journal and generally these are no different whether the writing (or representation) is on paper, screen or on an audio recorder, etc. There may be some 'effects' that can be utilized in electronic journals such as the allowance of a certain time period after the entry has been made for editing, after which the entry is permanent (for example, on WebCT). We make a brief reference to blogs at the end of this chapter.

More or less unstructured forms of journal

It is questionable whether any form of journal in a formal learning situation is truly unstructured. Any journal that will be overseen by another in authority is likely to be structured in accordance with the perceived expectations of the overseer. This hidden curriculum is of no mean significance as a structural influence. In unstructured forms of journal there is both free and reflecting writing – the subject matter and work in the journal is the choice of the writer, though it may be that the writer is expected to write in a specified regular manner, or to a certain length. It is possible that the writer will impose her own structure – as is illustrated in Chapter 13.

Structured forms of journals

By 'structure' we mean any imposed constraint on the way in which a journal is written. Structure can help students to obtain greater benefit from the journal. It can ensure that the learners reflect on the appropriate issues and can help them to 'move on' in their reflection and their learning. This may prevent them from 'going around in circles'. Structure may come in the form of themes for the form of writing – such as autobiography or recording that relates to a project or issue.

Autobiographical writing

There is an autobiographical element to the writing, perhaps in the way that previous events are related to the current time (e.g. as in Progoff, 1975). Such a form of writing may accompany a portfolio, providing a commentary on the materials in terms of personal development.

Double entry journals

In this type of journal, the recording of experience is first made in a descriptive manner. At a later time the writer reflects and writes further on the initial written account, drawing conclusions from it or at least 'moving it on'. This further writing may be spatially arranged alongside the original, sometimes on the opposite page to it. The secondary reflection that is involved in this system may be imposed by the format of the journal (as we have described above), or within the educational context by the imposition of an assessment task that requires further reflection on the initial reflective response or by a self-imposition. Shepherd found that he gained most from his journal if he went back over it and reflected further around three months after the first written account (Shepherd, 2004).

Structure is given as exercises

Some journals are substantially based on the provision of set activities or exercises such as those that are included in Chapter 13. There may, in addition, be some free writing.

Structure is given in the form of questions

Questions are posed calling for a response to or offering guidance on issues to be covered. A sequence of questions provides prompts that guide the learner to cover particular topics or the appropriate areas of material. The questions provided by Johns (1994) are an example here.

The journal is used to accompany other learning

The structure may be determined by other learning, which may be a programme of learning, a research project, or a placement, for example. The journal may be written in the planning stages if it accompanies a project. The entries may underpin reflection on what actual topic to choose for investigation as well as reflection on the events of the actual development. If the 'other learning' is a programme of learning, the learner may be asked to reflect, for example, on set reading, the content of lectures or seminars.

A journal format is used where the structure is provided within the journal itself

In this case the writers choose how to work within the set structure. Progoff's Intensive Journal is an example (see Chapter 13). In this case, the writers start writing in one section and move to another section, guided by the emerging themes as they work, or guided by what they want to explore. In the Intensive Journal there are suggested methods of working in the different sections.

Profiles or portfolios

There is another group of 'life accounts' that are not usually called journals', but can have the same effect. Portfolios tend to include other documents alongside sections of reflective writing which summarize and interelate the document content. There may also be graphic material, stories or poetry (see patchwork texts in Chapter 13). Profiles or portfolios are particularly common in professional development settings, in the accreditation of prior learning, in fieldwork and placements, and they are increasingly being used as a means of assessment in discipline-based higher education.

Dialogue journals and journals involved in communication between writers

We expand on the topic of dialogue journals here because the other forms of journal-writing will be described in later chapters. Dialogue journals are different from individually written journals in that they encourage the exchange and development of ideas between two or more writers. They can be like the exchange of letters or emails where the content is reflective and where there is an intention to increase learning. One writer starts, usually with a comment or a set of thoughts, and the journal with its entry is passed on to another who responds to the first, usually taking the ideas further, or adding new information. There are examples of this method in 'open' situations – such as among a group of students in a managed email discussion, or set in a context with the subject matter focused on the issues of that context – such as dialogue journals between teachers and their students or between teachers of a particular topic (Orem, 2001; Neopolitan, 2004; Chan and Chung, 2004; Rarieya, 2005).

Dialogue journals seem to have had their origins in school settings with young children corresponding with their teachers in the 1980s (Staton *et al.*, 1988), but their use is described in a number of contexts in more recent literature. These tend still to be in the teaching literature. Examples of their use are between professional teachers engaging in research of their practice (Roderick and Berman, 1984; Roderick, 1986) and between teacher educators and teaching students (Staton, 1988).

The literature on dialogue journals tends to make great claims for their advantages, but their purposes are not always very clear. Where they are used between an authority and a student, the former can steer the reflection of the latter in the conversation and the interaction is probably not unlike a tutorial. However, where the dialogue is between equals, the slow pace can have an effect of deepening thinking and learning and of allowing time for unexpected thoughts to contribute to the dialogue.

The modern parallel of the dialogue journal is the email conversation in newsgroups. As these groups tend to demonstrate, there is a need for someone to take on a role of managing a discussion so that it retains a focus or a stream, and perhaps of summarizing it from time to time. An interesting issue, which applies to any forms of journal that are word-processed, is whether the nature of the writing process is the same as that written on paper, or whether it is different. The speed of writing on a screen may be an initial difference as well as the ease of public viewing.

There are many different ways in which journals may be usefully shared. Cowan and Westwood (2004) were members of a group of higher education teachers who decided to subject themselves to what most of them set for students – the writing of a learning journal. The journals were reviewed by one of the group and 'facilitative comments' were made. As a result of the exercise, several of the group changed their manner of working with students, and several realized that the task which they were setting for their students was more demanding than they had realized (see also Alterio and McDrury, 2003).

A slightly different form of collaborative 'journal' (though it is not called a journal) is the 'jotter wallet' described by Longenecker (2002). The 'wallet' is a set of index cards that is held in turn by one of the group each week (in this case physicians on a medical postgraduate residency programme). The holder is asked to make notes on surprising or interesting cases, write summaries of 'meaningful patient or peer encounters', jot down ideas, inspirations, etc. The content of this is shared with the whole group weekly by the holder of the wallet who presents a case and poses a question that can focus group reflection and discussion, and then the wallet is passed to the next in turn.

Other variants of journal-writing

Web logs or blogs

We mentioned electronic methods of writing journals above, and said that, while the format is different, most of the principles that apply to paper-based journals apply similarly – and that is also the case with blogs. Blogs are an innovation that is likely to develop in educational use in the near future, and therefore it is worth giving a little more attention to the subject. A web log or blog is an internet site on which the written work and editing work of an individual or group is managed through a web browser. Because it is web-based, it is public and this does distinguish it from most other journal work. Similarly the ease of editing work on a screen distinguishes it from paper-based work. The blog may be added to at different times or by different people within a pre-determined group, and it is organized by the dates of the additions. There may be other information or links added into the accumulating material. There may be a search facility that can enable material within the blog to be located more easily.

In a small research study of blogs used in the context of media studies (Armstong *et al.*, nd), students said that they found the blogs which they had maintained a useful addition to their paper-based private 'notebooks'. The fact that the students were given time at the end of each class to add to their blog may have been crucial in their popularity – as the giving of time for writing of any kind of journal can be valuable. In the research, the students did not use the blogs for actual communication, though it was felt that the act of public display of their thinking and learning was important to them.

Thinkpoint

[Journal-writing] can be compare to the formation of a beautiful rainbow. A basic ingredient in both processes, the formation of a rainbow and the writing of a learning journal, is internal reflection. The kind of reflection the rainbow requires is defined by the laws of physics; the kind required for a learning journal is defined by learning theory ... Both processes ... rely on illumination by a strong light; the rainbow with illumination by the sun and the learning journal with illumination by the human mind. A rainbow is described as a set of coloured arcs seen against the sky, whereas a journal is a tapestry of events seen against a backdrop of human life. Both are pleasing, authentic and good.

(English and Gillen, 2001b)

Chapter 6

Journals in teaching and learning in higher education

Introduction

This chapter considers the applications of learning journals in formal educational settings. While the focus is higher education, much could apply also to the school situation. We deal with journals in subjects or disciplines mainly other than those in professional or vocational subjects which are covered in the next chapter. There is a large overlap in the two chapters, partly because the notion of reflection and reflective practice from professional education has been drawn into the currency of thinking in general higher education (e.g. Barnett, 1997).

The chapter is divided into two parts. The first part focuses on learning journals and reflective writing in more general activities of higher education that are not related specifically to a discipline – for example in personal development planning. The longer section reviews the place of learning journals in the context of learning in the disciplines in higher education. Within these two sections, there are many examples.

General applications of learning journals in higher education

In this section we draw together a range of initiatives in which activities are involved that generally meet the criteria for learning journals. An initiative may not be called a learning journal but may rely on some reflective writing which links theory, or more factual elements of writing, or the observation of real situations and represents a collection of material over time.

Personal development planning (PDP)

Personal development planning was introduced in the UK in *The Dearing Report* (NCIHE, 1997) as a part of the progress file that included the development of formal transcripts on which were detailed the achievements of the student, and a process that involved the student in forward planning and personal development work. The transcripts are largely a matter for institutional central record-keeping and PDP has developed mainly out of the two latter processes. Higher education institutions were expected to have mechanisms in place by the year 2005/6 and guidelines have been developed by the Quality Assurance Agency (QAA) to encourage this to occur. It is primarily a process for undergraduate students, though it is beginning to be used with postgraduates as well. The QAA definition of PDP is 'Structured and supported processes to develop the capacity of individuals to reflect upon their learning and achievement and to plan for their own personal education and career development' (QAA, 2000). One of the driving forces for PDP developments as far as Dearing was concerned was the observation either that graduates might know about their disciplines, but did not possess the kinds of skills that were required in employment, or that they actually did have ability in the skills, but did not have sufficient awareness of what they could do to engage in discussion about their skills. This was particularly evident at recruitment.

There are no prescribed methods for the running of the process of PDP – institutions just have to demonstrate that students are having the appropriate opportunities and experiences. Because PDP is essentially a personal process, in the end it is only the student who can choose to engage in it – or not. PDP experiences come, therefore, in many shapes and forms. Some PDP is run centrally and outside the modular structure – perhaps as part of the personal tutorial system. Within the modular system, PDP may be enacted in dedicated PDP modules (e.g. a careers skills module) or as an element in many modules – or institutions may map PDP across existing modules, demonstrating that the equivalent reflective activities are occurring anyway. Sometimes PDP is linked to specific experiences that students will be enabled to encounter – such as the reflection on a period of work experience.

The intention in this short account of PDP is to plot the role of learning journals or sometimes journal-type activities in what could be run as PDP. This will enable those involved in PDP developments to understand how to use this book – though we might say from the start that there is nothing in the work with learning journals that is not relevant to PDP in its various forms.

The various ways in which journals and journal activities may be linked to PDP are:

- where a kind of ongoing journal (electronic or handwritten) runs alongside a programme. It is not likely to be called a learning journal, but will actually fit our definitions of a journal in Chapter 1;
- where the maintenance of a journal contributes to the overall portfolio of PDP activities. The subject matter of the journal relates to PDP directly;
- where the maintenance of a journal contributes to the overall portfolio of PDP activities. The subject matter of the journal is discipline-based, but in the requirement of students to reflect, it is counted as a PDP activity as well;
- where the kinds of activities that might be used in a structured journal are designed into PDP. This book (and Cottrell 1999 and 2003; Moon, 2004a) provides many such exercises, which may be used several times over the period of a programme as the student progresses.

We elaborate on the first form of PDP – where a kind of ongoing journal – electronic or handwritten – runs alongside the programme, either a whole programme or part of one. In such cases, students would usually be provided with a format in which they are asked to reflect on various elements of their past, current and possible future plans. Periodically the student is asked to look at the programme and to fulfil various tasks that relate to the level of the student. At the beginning of a programme the issues may be a matter of generally settling into learning and surviving at university, of getting to know the systems and in particular, the appraisal and sources of support for necessary study skills. In the middle of an undergraduate programme, there is the need to help the student to think ahead in career terms and to think realistically about where she is achieving well and where there are 'gaps' that may be filled by extra effort. There may be schemes and systems (e.g. work experience) that will enable the student to gain extra capacities that will facilitate later employment. In the final year of a programme, the concerns will be on progress in dissertations or final examinations, and the realities of what happens next.

In this form of PDP, the student may be asked to appraise her current level of skills in communication, for example, via a specially designed form, and then perhaps to consider what she might do in order to raise her skills. There would usually be skills sessions linked to the PDP process. In some systems, this process will be linked to tutorial sessions. The student might, for example, be asked to produce a hard copy of the current PDP activities for her tutor and at an appointment with the tutor, be prepared to discuss the material. It is the experience of running systems that some students take to such activities with ease, and that others find an alien process. Some of the methods of introducing reflective activities which are presented later in this journal might have value in helping such students (and – sometimes – tutors too). Some universities have well developed systems of electronic PDP (Dunne, 2005). Paper-based PDP may follow a similar pattern. Cottrell provides a book-based version of exercises relevant to the different stages of a student programme (Cottrell, 2003).

Fieldwork or placement diaries/logs

Reflective writing, often in journals, is increasingly used as a means of accounting for and realizing learning in fieldwork, placements and in work experience. While it is generally recognized that students gain from the opportunity to engage in such experiences, the learning can be so varied and incoherent that it is difficult for the student to articulate it and apply it to other situations. Asking for written reflective accounts or journals that are either unstructured or structured in order to focus attention on particular aspects of the experience seems to be helpful. Students may have the opportunity to do work-experience modules which have a basis of reflective writing (e.g. Houghton, 1998). A variation on this theme in a practical setting, where some learning is formalized, is the use of journals to record incidental learning. An example of this is where dental students in clinics record the wealth of personal and incidental learning (Oliver, 1998). This might have particular relevance in situations where the stipulated learning is described in terms of competencies or national vocational qualifications.

Research or project journals

We have suggested earlier that journals can be a helpful adjunct to project work, forming a location for conventional activities. This writer would always develop a journal to accompany any major project such as the writing of a book. A journal can ensure that ideas, inspirations, the 'notes on the back of envelopes', contact details, the product of sessions of thinking or problem solving, as well as the feelings about the progress of the project (and so on) can be maintained in the same place – possibly within separate sections. From the experience of the writer, it may be necessary at some stage to number the pages and index the content of such a journal so that the material becomes accessible for later use. 'This process can be particularly useful where a number of people are involved in the work. It can then also be the focus for coordinating the group and for ensuring appropriate information flow and the sharing of ideas' (Hickman, 1987). We have cited examples of such project journals earlier (Shepherd, 2004; Glaze, 2002).

Career management work

Career management has become seen as more significant as part of the process of higher education – though often now it is included in personal development planning. It includes the development of career-seeking skills, the learning of employability skills, searching for a post and performing in interview and it is motivating and helpful if the activities are integrated. A journal, similar to the research or project journal, provides a location for noting achievements or experiences (e.g. the learning of skills) for deliberation and planning, and brings coherence to the process.

Lecture journals

The lecture journal is a general method of journal use that can cut across all disciplines in formal education and can be used alone or as a component of a disciplinary-based journal. One of the problems with the traditional lecture method is that in its usual form it may not provide the time during which learners can think about its content and relate that to previous learning or experience. Students also often feel the need to take notes during lectures, which may further cut down the opportunity for taking a deep approach to learning (Chapter 2). It is probably fair to say that most students collect the notes from the day's classes and file them away for later reference. A lecture journal, however, in which they reflect on the content of a lecture, provides the opportunity to deepen and thereby to improve the quality of learning. The lecturer may manage the situation –

learners might, for example, be asked to formulate a series of questions that arise from the content of the lecture or to record a conversation with another about the lecture.

The development of writing skills

The ability to write is a necessary skill that most graduates would be expected to possess – and yet there is continuous comment about deficits in such skills (Lea and Stierer, 2000; Lea and Street, 2000). Within the current initiatives on widening participation, we have learners engaging in higher education who have written no more than a shopping list for many years – and perhaps who have never written an essay (Moon, 2005b). Journal-writing does seem to improve written self-expression and, on this basis, provides another means of bringing writing into higher education – particularly into disciplines such as mathematics, where it might not normally feature. As the second section in this chapter indicates, however, there are other reasons for instituting journals within disciplines such as mathematics.

In adult education or for those returning to education

Because journals are a means of identifying, raising awareness of, and accounting for learning, they have value for those in adult education or who are returning to education (Christensen, 1981; English and Gillen, 2001b). Sometimes these uses of journals are no different from those in any other higher education situation – sometimes they have specific roles for older learners. Redwine (1989), for example, describes the use of reflective autobiographical writing with students attending a ten-day orientation seminar prior to engagement in a degree programme based on distance learning and she identifies a number of roles that the writing fulfils. It is cathartic, helping students to bring to the fore and to deal with parts of their life histories – 'adults enter or re-enter the educational cycle with needs and characteristics that are very different from those of 18–22 year olds' (1989: 89). The shared writing develops group support that can persist and the task underpins the development of claims for credit for prior learning. Redwine's work takes account of the fact that adults returning to education have more experience to integrate with the new material of learning (Chapter 2) and a journal can have advantages to them in a manner that would not be reflected in the same way for those in their teens (Hiemstra, 2001; Boud, 2001).

Journals in the disciplines

While subject groups and headings are used to organize the content of this section, many of the techniques can be applied in other disciplinary contexts. Similarly, across the accounts below, practically all purposes for writing journals (Chapter 5) are represented explicitly or as an outcome.

The sciences, engineering and mathematics

This is a group of subjects in which journal-writing might appear not to have a place. However, among a relatively few accounts in the literature, there are clear indications of the manner in which journal-writing can facilitate learning and help with writing and there are some descriptions of useful techniques.

Perhaps the most helpful reports are those that are experimental. Selfe *et al.* (1986) studied the manner in which journal-writing could help mathematics students. Initially their intention was to compare the test grades of a group that was asked to write journals with another group using traditional methods. They found, however, that the influence of journal-writing was more subtle. The general finding in the initial investigation was that journal-writing was no better or worse than activities involving testing or quizzes at promoting learning. On a subsequent investigation, journals appeared to facilitate learning in a number of ways. By allowing them to think in a manner that was their own and to use their own language, the students were able to develop personal conceptual definitions that were much more understandable than technical definitions. The concrete nature of this thinking facilitated comprehension and application of abstract concepts and they began to evaluate or appreciate the usefulness of the concepts. The other two effects relate to the ability to solve problems. There was evidence in the writing that students were recording strategies which they found helpful in problem solving. Furthermore, in writing about problems instead of just working on calculation, they were coming to solutions through the writing. An excerpt from the writing of one student illustrates well the last point: 'I see nothing in common with the three functions except that the derivative has a power of N–i just like all the other derivatives have. Oh – wait a see, now I see how you did it. You took the derivative of the first term and . . .' (Selfe *et al.*, 1986: 200). It is interesting to see the same process evident in the writing of much younger students (age 11) (Mayher *et al.*, 1983).

Selfe also worked with engineering students (Selfe and Arbabi, 1986), with a primary intention of introducing more writing into the course. The students, in a structural analysis and design class, were asked to write at least a page a week on their experiences of the course. While their initial reaction was negative, and for a few (around 10 per cent) it remained negative, most found that 'it helped . . . [them to] clarify their thoughts, work out strategies for solving engineering problems, understand the important aspects of the structures course and identify areas in which they needed more help' (1986: 185). In contrast to a control group, those who had written in journals wrote final reports that 'were generally more coherent, organized and complete with better description of methods used to solve engineering problems'. Instructors also felt much more informed about their students' processes of learning. Gibbs (1988) describes the use of journals in engineering in a somewhat similar manner.

Two examples of journal-writing in physics broadly parallel the observations above. Jensen (1987) describes the use of journals initially in order to improve writing among physics students. His students wrote on assigned topics at the beginning, in the middle or at the end of lecture sessions for seven or eight minutes and they were encouraged to reflect personally. Some of the topics were: 'Explain to your mother why water stays in a pail when swung in a vertical circle around your head' or 'Discuss the net effect of leaving the fridge door open'. Jensen observes that the writing was initially formal and textbook-like and then became freer, exploring and extrapolating. Jensen suggests that the value seems not so much that the students had the opportunity to write, but that they were 'thinking on paper'. It is worth reiterating a comment in Chapter 2 suggesting that the requirement to be able to explain seems likely to encourage a deep approach to learning.

Grumbacher (1987) focused on the ability of physics students to solve problems. She observed the writing processes of students whom she considered to be good problem solvers. They articulate the problems clearly, use visualization and verbalization in the solving and they are aware of the relative appropriateness of their responses. More significantly 'they use their learning logs to synthesize their new knowledge about physics with their prior knowledge and experiences' (1987: 325). On the basis of the map of reflective writing, they move through the reflective thinking process. Grumbacher suggests that other students can 'learn the process good problem solvers follow by practicing the process in logs or journals' (1987: 326) From her reflections on how journals help physics students, Grumbacher also suggests that journals encourage students to initiate questions, and that once they have posed a question, they are inclined to work in order to answer them. She considers that journals help to provide the opportunity for students to 'play with the ideas of physics' in order better to understand. Perhaps this has similarities to the work with journals done by students on a Master's level programme in Environmental Studies – where one intention for the project management log was to enable students to develop a sense of ownership of their academic work (Stephani et al., 2000).

Another form of journal in science subjects is the report. We described the research of McCrindle and Christensen (1995) on report writing in biology in Chapter 2. The research was focused more on the learning from the journals than on the quality of communication, but it could well be argued that the greater understanding and metacognitive ability that were achieved by the journal-writing group are likely to contribute to the quality of reports.

Observation is relevant to report writing in science. Fulwiler (1986) describes how journal-writing 'teaches people to see better . . . I begin to look at the world differently because I know I will write about it because writing about anything causes me to notice it more fully'. He describes a use of a 'notebook' in biology in which students are asked not only to record what they see but also what they think about what they see. Writing informally, he suggests, they see better and better understand what they see. Wilkinson describes the use of journals for electronics and engineering students for a similar requirement (Wilkinson and Robb, nd).

Journals may provide means for communication between students and with the tutor (e.g. as in the dialogue journal described in Chapter 5), but DiBiase (1999) provides useful information about what he calls a 'travelling' journal used in a science methods class. The journal contains comments, thoughts and reflections and questions and in a pattern that he describes, it travels between students and their tutors – and, he says, it 'forces you to think'. Usefully, DiBiase provides some assessment criteria.

English and allied subjects

There are many ways of using journals in the subject areas that make up English and drama. Several utilize the freer forms of self-expression as a means of improving other more formal academic writing. Flynn (1986) used journals in English alongside a text as a means of increasing students' understanding of the text. The response to a literary text shifts from 'expression to transaction, from reader orientated to writer orientated' (1986: 209). Students were asked to write their personal responses to a particular text in journals and then to write a first draft of their account of the text. Flynn describes the first draft typically as too involved in the text and unfocused. In the final draft, the reader learns to view the text from a greater distance, seeing details that he or she has previously missed. Flynn argues that it is important for time to be spent in the exploratory phase, with written products being the result of an 'extended process of discovery' (1986: 213). She says 'pedagogical structures which encourage students to read and to write in stages also encourage them to transform their perceptions of texts which, in turn, may encourage them to transform their perceptions of their worlds and of themselves' (1986: 213).

Lindberg (1987) applies the use of journals in a manner different from that of Flynn to achieve a similar objective – of helping learners to gain a deeper understanding of texts. He uses a dialectical (or double entry) journal. Students write their observations of and reactions to the text on one side of the page. These may include 'times when your reading changes you are surprised or puzzled something just does not fit . . . your first impression of the ending'. When the story is read, they are asked to go back and make sense of the observations. These journals are discussed in a planned series of 'conferences'.

Gatlin (1987), again working with literary texts, started out with the anticipation of successful deep learning from journal work but reports how he failed to persuade his students to work comfortably and independently in journals. The situation, however, reversed when he began to share his own journal-writings with his class. 'The result was dramatic because the rest of the class not only experienced a real example of a journal entry but they began to regard me as a fellow learner, not just an authority figure. This broke some thick ice in the class and brought about a real improvement in their journals and in our class discussions' (1987: 112).

Tama and Peterson (1991) use literary texts for a different, almost opposite, purpose to those above. While journals in the paragraphs above facilitate learning about the text and literature, these writers describe the use of journals in mediating learning about self from the reading of literature. Tama and Peterson select a group of texts around a theme such as the character of teachers – and through reading and reflecting in journals, students learn – or 'weigh and consider' as they quote from Francis Bacon – how it is to be a teacher. Learning about a role is carried to a greater extreme in the example of journal use given by Craig from an example in drama (Dillon, 1983). Sister Craig describes how children (in this case) learned to become more secure in their roles in a drama production by writing a daily journal in role.

We have described how Lindberg uses double entry journals to help students to understand meaning in a literary text. Joyce (nd) uses a similar format in information skills classes to help students to evaluate sources of information. The page is divided into two. The students are asked to read an article or a chapter of a book, to read some quotations and to summarize or to respond to the material on one side of the journal. On the other side, they evaluate the material in terms of authenticity, currency, bias or overt point of view, reliability and so on. The journal entries support a discussion and students are asked to write up their discussion in their journals. Kent (1987) lays a few groundrules to guide students on the use of journals in an introduction to philosophy course. In 'free writing', they are told to write what they like, but they must present the views of the subject accurately and logically. They are required to support any judgements they might make about the views. Kent suggests that the success of journals in his large class is that they exploit formal academic writing and informal self-expressive writing – and that for a subject like philosophy it is necessary to function in both.

In recent years there has been a substantial increase in creative writing subjects in higher education. There are examples of the use of journals to enhance creative writing in the literature. Lipman (2003) talks of maintaining a story journal to enhance the 'story mind' and much of Hunt's work is relevant to journal-writing, although it is not specifically written for that purpose. As Chapter 11 will indicate, story and journal-writing become intertwined – and may often enhance each other (Moon, 2004a).

The humanities and social sciences

Wagenaar introduced a journal in sociology in order to encourage students to relate the theory taught on the course to their own observations and experiences for the purposes of meeting 'the higher level cognitive objectives in her or his course' (Wagenaar, 1984). He describes it as 'an intellectual exercise in reflexivity' which exploits the functions of evaluation and application (Bloom, 1956). Students were not asked to write about their feelings but from the examples given, feelings were present and acceptable in their expressions. The process of journal-writing was relatively simple. Two elements were to be present in the journal – the observation of behaviour and the discussion in theoretical terms. There were two formats in which the students could write. They could either describe the observation and then relate it to theory – or they could combine the two. Wagenaar suggests that there are a number of areas of sociology where journal-writing of this kind is helpful, and he cites Jensen (1979) who asked students to focus on one topic in the area of social problems in their journals for a term. The narrowing of the subject matter allows a wider range of consideration. For example, students could follow the topic in professional journals as well as in the popular press.

Steffens (1987) advocates the use of journals in history classes for a similar purpose to Wagenaar. He wants the journal entries to provide a link between experiences and existing knowledge and the history topic in hand. In discussing the role of writing in history, he points out that history does not exist without writing, 'doing history means writing history' (1987: 219). He acknowledges the importance of writing as communication but suggests that there is a further role, albeit one that is not as frequently exploited. Writing informally 'provides an opportunity to develop ideas, to "see" those ideas and to decide whether they disagree or agree with themselves . . . We know a great deal more history than we can usually recall immediately' (1987: 219). He suggests that exploratory writing provides time and space for students to relate theory and new knowledge to what they discover that they know already.

In this form of journal, students were asked to write entries on a given topic in class and at home, interrelating the inputs and providing a personal response in the form of questions, speculation and doubts. Questions and tasks were used to generate ten minutes of writing at the beginning of a class. To illustrate their diversity, some examples of the questions/tasks for the topic European Cultural History, 1880–1930 are:

> 'Vienna of the 1890s has been stigmatized as the training ground of Adolph Hitler. Was Paris of the 1890s any different?'

> 'What is the most interesting thing I have come to so far in my research paper?' (The research was a required task.)

> 'List all the things for which Einstein is famous.'

Steffens also describes the use of journal entries to draw conclusions at the end of a class. Brodsky and Meagher (1987) use a similar approach to journals in political science. One of the features of the teaching strategy was to ask students to complete some entries on assigned tasks and a given number of entries on a subject matter of their choice. Evaluations of learning taking place in classes were also included. The journals were used as a means of initiating classroom discussion. Baltensperger (1987), working with geography students, describes a similar element in his work with classroom journals. He posed a question to students and asked them to write their responses first. He would then ask the question again, requesting oral reports based on the written ideas, and then would open the discussion for more general comment. He found this a valuable means of combating problems of poor response to oral questions posed in class.

There are a number of reports on journals in psychology in the literature, with those by Hettich probably the best known. In two papers, separated by 14 years, Hettich advocated similar functions for journals in psychology – similar as well to the purposes advocated by Wagenaar (above) (Hettich, 1976, 1990). Journals were seen to help students to connect course learning to their real experiences and observations. The emphasis is on the course material, and instructions indicated that entries could contain 'examples that show comprehension of the concept; application or experimentation with principles; and analysis, evaluation and synthesis of course concepts' (Hettich, 1990). Journals were used in a different manner in a course in adolescent psychology (McManus, 1986). While they still served to relate theory to practice, an important part of the students' learning in practice focused on a series of regular meetings of the college students with local adolescents. The journals charted the learning from the experience of the meetings. Another example of journal use in psychology is most unusual. Terry (1984) asked students to record instances of forgetting during the period of the course on memory. They were required to write the situation, the activities in which they were engaged and their emotional state and to consider the factors involved in forgetting and retrieval.

In a project to investigate the impact of different forms of writing in anthropology, Creme (1998) describes three different forms of journals in a social anthropology department. Project logs accompanied a first-year course that introduced the theoretical and conceptual basis to anthropology research. The logs were used in a research project and contained recordings and reflection on the records. The second form is called a record of study. Students developed an account of their learning from different sources throughout the course with a focus on the development of 'understanding of central course concepts'. The third form of journal was used in a first-year multidisciplinary course on death. In their journals, students explored their reactions to various accounts of death and to their personal experiences.

Languages

Mülhaus and Löschmann (1997) discuss issues relating to foreign language learning in modularized higher education. The change from integrated programmes to the accumulation of modules means that students enrolling on a module are likely to have diverse backgrounds in relation to the subject matter. A distance learning approach was adopted with students using workshop time for advice and progress checks. With this approach, the writers considered that students needed to give attention to their learning strategies and they used journals to address that need. Journals included the written work of students – video summaries, vocabulary lists, worksheet tasks and self-reflective comments. A marking scheme assessed 'the interaction with the material and the depth of the learning process as evident from the students' vocabulary lists, translations and comments' (1997: 25). The comments on learning made in the journals both formed the basis of workshops and were shared for others to try.

There are aspects in common between the approach above and that of Finch (1998). Finch used journals with 'false beginners': Korean students needing language skills to cope both with learning in English and needing new skills and confidence to cope with the cultural differences in learning. Finch's journal was very structured, with questionnaires for completion about skills and attitudes in language learning, self-evaluation forms and a blank section for personal reflections.

English, of course, is also a foreign language to many and there are examples both to support the learning to teach element of the process, as well as a tool in the classroom processes to support students who are learning English as a future medium for study. Tsang (2003) used journals with non-native pre-service teachers of English as a second language and found that it enabled them to become more critically reflective. Orem (2001) describes the use of journals in this context in more general terms (in adult education), and supplies other useful references. He says,

> There does appear to be widespread agreement that improved practice can result from ongoing personal reflection on practice. Practicing adult educators can be encouraged to make reflection a regular part of their own professional development programme. Second language learners can be encouraged to reflect on their learning as they develop their language skills. In both cases, journal-writing can provide the vehicle for reflection that leads to more effective pactice.
>
> (Orem, 2001: 76–7)

Arts subjects

The first three examples in this section on journals in arts subjects may look the same, but they have different purposes. One form of journal that is a natural accompaniment to the creation of music and drama is the project type of journal where the development of ideas is recorded and considered reflectively in the journal. The aim is to enhance the thought processes that contribute to the project. With art and design students, Davies (1998) set a similar journal that accompanies project work, but where the main aim is one of assessment. He suggests that there can be too much focus on the outcome of art student work and not on the all-important process of it. The journals demonstrate process, and assessment is on this basis. A third example of journal that may coincide with those above is a journal that itself generates creative ideas. Rainer's (1978) many ideas for types of journal include the development of what she calls 'a sourcebook for creative projects'.

The fourth example in this section is different. Ambrose (1987) describes a music journal. Like many others, initially the journal was a means of improving writing. Students were asked to write their comments about concerts attended, music heard and books read about music. However, the journals served the purpose of monitoring the students' listening behaviour. They were expected, for example, to attend a certain number of concerts. Ambrose observed that the written work of students improved.

Business and law

Business subjects range from number-based to literary studies though the social sciences of management and leadership. November (1993) makes a comment about his subject, commerce, that may apply quite widely in this range of subjects. He suggests that the study environment is not always conducive to deep approaches to learning (Chapter 2). He used journals in order to deepen the quality of learning in a final-year course. Over the time that he used this method, he found that the best results occurred when considerable guidance on the journal-writing was given. One method that he reports is to ask students to write an 'agenda' – a list of problems or issues of concern, and then to examine each in a systematic manner. Every so often he asked students to review the kinds of questions that are raised in their writing.

Both Wolf (1980) and Ficher (1990), using journals for administration and marketing studies respectively, indicate that an important purpose of the method is the provision of a means of linking the classroom learning with the business world. Wolf's instructions to students were to focus on a 'moment or event' from four perspectives. The first is outer experience (as a third-person description), the next is one of reflection and generalization to deepen understanding, the third stage is 'inner experience' (a subjective account), and the fourth is more reflection and generalization to connect the current focus with previous experiences. There is an 'appendix' which represents a periodic overview of themes and agendas for future learning. This work was based on the Kolb cycle (Kolb, 1984).

Ficher's students were asked to make one journal entry per class, relating 'real world' observations to the class material, using the correct terminology. The recognition of this relationship was the first purpose which journals were to fulfil. Another was to 'increase student sensitivity to consumer behaviour', a third was to increase participation in the class and the fourth was to improve oral and written communication skills. Elkins (1985) describes the use of journals in the context of law. The journals were a means of counteracting the uncaring and subject-centred attitudes that he describes in legal education. In the journals 'legal education is presented . . . as it is personally experienced, as individual students "see" it, "feel" it, and make it part of their lives'. Perhaps the idea that journals contribute in any subject to 'making it part' of the student's life is a reminder that most of the applications of journals in the different subjects that are mentioned above apply far more broadly. With a bit of thought they can facilitate learning in different ways in many contexts.

There are a number of reports on journal-writing in the context of management training. We have mentioned Shepherd (2004) whose personal journal, written as he developed into the role of a volunteer management advisor in Cambodia, provides useful insights for journals set in fieldwork in management education. In addition, Rothwell and Ghelipter (2003) raise many practical issues as well as making useful observations of journal work with a group of Israeli students. Their work was based on students in undergraduate degrees in management – on work with more than 6,000 students over a period of time. Unlike many reports, they were concerned with the quality of reflective work done by the students and raise the issue of depth and levels (see Chapter 4). Betts also raises questions about reflective practice in management education – asking if it is 'Theology, therapy or picket line', that is, asking what it means that something is being done in a particular way (Betts, 2004: 244). She describes the use of journals with learners, and analyses the nature of the content in these three terms, concluding that 'some teachers should take a more critical view of the purposes for and the outcomes of journals. We refer further to the work mentioned here in Chapter 9 (in the context of ethical issues).

Kallaith and Coghlan (2001) used journals in a graduate programme in organization development and change. They report that the students generally found the journals useful, the highest ratings being for the manner in which journals enabled the learners to relate theory to 'real life' and how they enabled learners to integrate the new knowledge. It is interesting to note the name of 'change journal' that was employed for this work.

Thinkpoint

In the ordinary way, our sense of identity depends upon interaction with the physical world and with other people. My study, lined with books, reflects my sense of what kind of person I consider myself to be. My relationships with my family, with colleagues, friends, and less intimate acquaintances, define me as a person who holds certain views and who may be expected to behave in ways which are predictable . . . But I may come to feel that such habitually defining factors are also limiting. Suppose that I become dissatisfied with my habitual self or feel that there are areas of experience or self-understanding which I cannot reach. One way of exploring these is to remove myself from present surroundings and see what emerges . . . Removing oneself voluntarily from one's habitual environment promotes self-understanding and contact with those inner depths of being which elude one in the hurly-burly of day to day life.

(Storr, 1988: 34–5)

Chapter 7

Journals in professional education and development

Introduction

This chapter concerns the use of journals in professional education and professional development. The chapter refers to journals in the beginning stage of professional education as well as in practising professional stages, often in the form, then, of a professional portfolio. The chapter is divided into five sections. The first concerns journals that are orientated towards the development of the self as a professional. The second section concerns journals that improve practice, often by making the link between theory and practice. The next section concerns journals that focus on professional empowerment by raising and working with socio-political awareness. The penultimate section reviews examples of the ways in which journals can support elements of educational programmes. The last section is based on one specific example of a journal used in a multi-professional manner with professionals from a number of different professions. As we have said before, however, most journals are set for or fulfil several purposes and that is the case with many journals in this chapter. We have not made a division between practising professionals and novices. In this age of learning across the lifetime, there is a sense that education and development are continuous – only the content and methods may vary.

It may also be difficult to draw the line between journals used in academic disciplines (described in the previous chapter) and vocational development as there are elements of professional education that are subject orientated and aspects of subject-orientated learning that are common to professional development learning. Engineering students become engineers as much as education students become teachers and yet the former tend to be seen as less vocational than the latter. Similarly many professional journals address self-development (next chapter).

When the first edition of this book was written, journals were much more prevalent in nursing and education and speculation as to why this should be suggested that reflection seemed to be so much a part of the ethos of these professions and both have tended to be more commonly taken up by women who may be more reflective by nature (Clarke *et al.*, 1996). Both professions rely on interpretive knowledge which is socially constructed and not rooted in a body of 'fact' (Schön, 1987). Both also rely on decisions made 'on the spot' with unpredictable situations being relatively common. Action is what counts but the consequences of action can be critical.

Whatever is the truth of the reasoning about the professional origins of journal-writing, the use of reflection and journals are much more widespread. The rationales for journal practice in different professions is often similar, though there may be specific features that characterize the profession. Teacher education students are often asked to explore their own experiences of being in school (see below) and the journals of nurses seem to be more orientated towards the nature of their interaction with patients (Landeen *et al.*, 1992). A general characteristic of professional development journals is their willingness to address past, present and the anticipation of future practice – not just present action.

Journals in the development of self as a professional

We have commented on the notion that professional development often involves self-development. This is more likely to be particularly the case in professions where the nature of the activity demands a response from the whole person. To facilitate learning or to nurture educational development involves the whole person cognitively and emotionally – and a similar scenario is true of the art of patient care. Because most journal-writing draws expression or exploration of emotion and attitude into the 'open' in writing, it has the potential to link personal and professional education and development. Additionally, with the role of emotions and attitudes recognized, there is an unusually good possibility of examination and possible modification. Where they can remain hidden, the opportunity for change is limited.

In the context of the development of self as a professional, a number of writers talk of the development of 'voice'. Oberg and Underwood (1992) wrote a joint paper in which they describe the dialogue journal between them, one as teacher educator and one as student (Underwood). The accounts describe Underwood finding her 'inner voice', her 'own tale in the telling'. In this process, she recognized herself as 'becoming . . . whole, both the creator and interpreter of meaning'. Canning (1991), however, notes the later reflections of qualified teachers who also felt that they were finding a 'voice' in their reflective processes, but they suggested that the potential 'voice' of students is often subdued by their training 'to please, to defer to professors and supervisors for good grades and positive evaluations'. Others of Canning's group felt that their voices were thwarted by mechanistic attitudes to the teaching process by administrators. One of her subjects rationalized: 'I may not be able to change decisions . . . but now I know what I'm thinking.'

Wolf (1989) illustrates the use of the metaphor of voice in journals in the education of gerontologists. Her aim was to counteract the tendency of the literature and theory of ageing to 'objectify' and distance the ageing process. Her concern is that students will consider that older people are 'out there' rather than a part of themselves. She talks about the focus that the journal gives to encouraging students to hear the inner voice, to 'open up', to articulate the fears of ageing. She says: 'In learning to articulate our inner voice, we must focus on ourselves; the act of composing our thoughts in journal form helps shape this activity.'

Strengthening 'voice' and increasing comfort in professional situations are among a mass of qualities that are related to journal-writing which amount, in general terms, to increasing confidence in the professional role. Ashbury et al. (1993) used journals in a communications course with first-year students in medicine. Here the emphases were on the development of confident communications with potential patients, personal reflection and evaluation of the course experience. Ashbury et al. comment that the students' journals enabled them to become aware:

> of many of the concerns and struggles of medical students as they progressed through first year issues . . . [The] students identified and addressed issues related to their future role as doctors, their suitability for that career, the effect of their gender on that role, patients' perceptions of doctors . . . and the complexities of communication, interviewing and learning in small groups.
>
> (Ashbury et al., 1993)

Among others reporting on this development of confidence are, for teaching students, Dart et al. (1998) and Rovegno (1992) and, for nurses, Dimino (1988).

Another type of journal focuses more deliberately on the progression through and recording of the experiences of developing professionals. What is termed 'journal' here might there be called by such terms as portfolio, a professional profile or record of achievement (James and Denley, 1993). Such documents may play a large part in the assessment of the course or may be used to assess the professional for probationary periods or for promotion. The reflective writing element in them may be less important as a means of learning, and more important as a means of linking the elements of the portfolio into a more coherent presentation (Paulson et al., 1991). It is worth noting that, while the examples we have given above are developed concurrently with the accumulation of the experiences, a portfolio may be developed from past recorded experiences, as in the case of the accreditation of prior learning or PhDs by presentation of a portfolio of work.

Autobiography has often had a role within professional development journal-writing. Autobiography is also retrospective and may form an exercise (Knowles, 1993) with a major use in teacher education. The assumption is that during childhood contacts with learning, school and teachers, a range of emotions, attitudes, understandings and personal beliefs develop about the educational situation. Along the lines of constructivist thinking, these 'personal theories' (Griffiths and Tann, 1992), represented in the cognitive structure of students (Chapter 2), form the basis for professional learning. The elements of prior learning are likely to be represented as 'knowledge-in-pieces' – a relatively incoherent foundation on which to build a future teacher's orientation to his or her profession (Winitzky and Kauchak, 1997). Making this knowledge, emotion and attitude explicit allows them to be examined and related constructively to new learning. A journal is an ideal vehicle for this exercise since it can provide present and anticipated future contexts alongside working in the past and it can provide the opportunities to return to past experiences on many different occasions.

Experiences of autobiographical journal exercises suggests that the context of the present is influential on the nature of memories that emerge on any particular occasion (Aspinwall, 1986). To take account of this phenomenon, Grumet (1987) recommends the use of the currere technique (after Pinar, 1975) in which the past, present and future anticipations of an experience are considered at the same time (see Chapter 13). In a later paper, Grumet suggests that it is not just the writing part of the process that is important, but the reading of the accounts as well. She says:

> Reading autobiography invites its reader to discriminate the particular from the general in her own account. It makes it possible to ground an approach to pedagogy in what she has known and experienced without requiring her to impose her experience on the students. It invites the individual to attend to the differences as well as to the similarities between the world in which she came to form and the worlds that her students come from.
>
> (Grumet, 1989)

Grumet goes on to suggest that a further stage of working with autobiography can be the critical consideration of the material from the perspectives of educational philosophy, psychology, sociology and history. She sees this process as linking the realm of private thought to that of public knowledge so that the validity of personal thought processes is recognized and becomes a part of professional education and development.

Journals in the development of practice

Perhaps the most common use of journals in professional education is in the context of practice or in moving between classroom theory and situations of practice (Brookfield, 1995). This is a process that is superficially similar to that described in the previous chapter where students made better sense of their theory in the disciplines by linking it to common events in 'the real world' (e.g. Hettich, 1990). However, in the professional context the emphasis is not always on the development of more sound theory, but more often on the enhancement of practice. This is particularly relevant in the face of political pressure to make – teacher training, for example – more practical and relevant (Griffiths and Tann, 1992).

Dart et al. (1998) studied the way in which graduate trainee teachers used their journals as a means of relating theory to practice. In the early part of their one-year course, students would comment on theory and not relate it to practice situations ('no connection'). At a later stage a second form of link between theory and practice emerged. Here theory was used to inform practice and generally the reverse of this did not occur at that time. The examples of student journal comments suggest that students were demonstrating this in practical situations or in metacognitive comments about their own learning. An example of the former is of a student who recognized that a teacher is not 'a provider of knowledge' but a 'facilitator of learning' and then goes on to suggest to herself ways of facilitating learning in order to 'make things relevant and enjoyable'. An example of the latter is where a student comments on how her use of concept maps was helpful to her methods of learning. Later still in the course, Dart *et al.* observed some journal entries that demonstrate both theory-to-practice and practice-to-theory links.

Journals have also been used to support reflective practice – both in its development and in its function. However, there is a difficulty in generalizing in these areas because 'reflective practice' has different meanings and connotations. In an interesting metaphor, Wellington (1991) described the qualities of reflective practice as those of a 'tenacious' city wild flower which 'vibrates with vitality, raising our awareness and calling us from passivity into action'. In somewhat less colourful language, we have described reflective practice as a set of abilities and skills with a focus on the taking of a critical stance (see next section in this chapter), an orientation to problem solving or a state of mind (Moon, 1999b). Journals have a role in the development of all of these capacities and attitudes as the following comments and examples continue to indicate.

The instructions for journal-writing for reflective practice vary. In some examples of the use of journals, the instruction has been to reflect freely, and in others, structure is imposed in a variety of manners. In an example of the former, Hoover (1994) describes the journals of two teaching students. One made satisfactory use of the journal to make sense of his practical experiences. The other, however, increasingly used her journal to work out her 'identity crisis' with regard to teaching and she eventually left the programme. It is a moot point as to whether the journal performed a useful task for the latter student. Hoover indicates that she did not see this as a successful use of journal activities and that more structure could have guided writing into 'deliberations about educational principles and practice'.

In a relatively simple example of structure in journals used to generate reflective practice, Sparkes-Langer *et al.* (1990) describe a journal assignment in which they asked students each day to describe one successful and one less successful event of the day. The students were asked to consider the context and issues raised, and focus on 'why' questions about the events. Another relatively simple structure was given as an option by Francis (1995). Teaching students were asked initially to describe an event ('a brief summary of the key points'), to indicate new insights that came out of the session, then to consider emerging questions and to provide a personal reaction.

In keeping with the work on quality and depth in reflection (Chapter 4), Morrison (1996) is concerned that teaching students 'move on' in their thinking through journals. He bases his work with journals and other means of encouraging reflective practice on two models. In the first model, the reflection is directed towards the actions of the student. It uses Schön's (1983) notions of 'reflection-in-action' and 'reflection-on-action', and poses questions to help students in their reflection. Students are asked, for example, to consider their personal, professional, academic and evaluative development in such areas as increasing knowledge, attitudinal changes and 'the expansion (in depth and breadth) of their vision'. In the second part of the model, reflection is seen more in terms of empowerment and political awareness. Such considerations, as we have suggested earlier, have the potential to deepen reflective activity. Issues concerning the functioning of the self in a particular setting (Prawat, 1991) are related to the experiences of the students in their strands of development.

In the field of nursing, Johns (1994) provides a list of questions that can guide the learning from experience. Like Morrison, the first questions encourage the description of the experience. The next section is headed 'Reflection'. In it he proposes questions such as 'What was I trying to achieve?', 'What were the consequences of my action for myself, the patient/family, the people I work with?' and three further questions about the feelings of himself, the patient, and 'How do I know how the patient felt about it?' He brings in 'Influencing factors' of a personal (internal) nature and external nature and queries what sources of knowledge 'did/should have influenced my decision-making?' The last questions that Johns recommends concern the learning that emerges from the process of reflection – any changes in feelings, proposed changes in behaviour or under-standing of wider issues (e.g. ethics).

Heath's (1998) work is also in the field of nursing and, as we have indicated earlier, she proposes the use of double entry journals. A valuable aspect of her use of journals is the recognition of the need for different forms of guidance for those more advanced in the profession or more able at reflective writing. The general pattern of this progression is from the simplest form of reflection in which the practitioner realizes that practice is an important source of learn-ing and knowledge. At the next stage there is recognition that the learning has implications for future practice and there is some linking of theory and practice. At the most advanced stage, there is a broadening and deepening of the content of reflection.

Stuctured and free formats have their roles in journal-writing. Structured journals support practice and help a student to make sense of the experiences; however, in the new and challenging situations of learning or working in a pro-fession, the free-writing areas of journals can act with all the qualities of purely personal journals. They can act as 'friend', somewhere to vent feelings, to note new enthusiasms or to sort out the daily new dilemmas and difficulties – or to generate material to be dealt with in a more structured manner.

Journals used to develop socio-political awareness

We have mentioned above a few writers who have included socio-political or ethical reasoning in journal tasks and we commented that dealing with these issues can be an effective manner of deepening the reflection process. A few other writers, however, have focused directly on the development of critical awareness of this kind. Sparkes-Langer and Colton (1991) distinguish the development of critique by suggesting that cognitive elements of reflection 'emphasize how teachers make decisions', but 'the critical approach stresses the substance that drives the thinking: the experiences, beliefs, sociopolitical values and goals . . .'. Proponents of this approach have been, for example, Smyth (1987) and Tripp (1987). Smyth observes the 'skills-related way in which most in-service education had been conceived and enacted'. He sees work of this sort on teacher improvement as 'intellectually bankrupt'. He considers that what is important is to 'challenge the myth that somehow classroom teaching is, or should be, a detached, neutral . . . and value-free activity'. The work on which Smyth based this was with a group of teachers involved in 'active critique and an uncovering of the tensions that exist between particular teaching practices and the larger cultural and social contexts in which teaching is embedded'. By working in a group, and using journals to record classroom incidents, they sought to move beyond the technical interpretations of the social settings of classrooms as representing the source of limitations on teaching. They re-evaluated these sources of limitation as elements in a system in which any 'rules, roles and structures' could potentially be challenged.

A description of the incidents was the first of four stages in developing the critique. The second stage questioned first the meaning behind the teaching ('informing'). This involved seeking theories that lay behind the description of the event or relationships between elements in it. The 'reconstructing' phase concerned the manner in which the event might have been handled differently, and the 'confronting' phase considers the assumptions, beliefs and values that underlie events, the manner in which they are maintained, and whose interest they serve.

Smyth's work was undertaken with practising teachers; however, the principles of it are applied in teacher education. There is some question as to whether student teachers are sufficiently knowledgeable to challenge the system into which they move (Moon, 1999b).

We have mentioned Stockhausen and Kawashima's work with Japanese nurses (2002). It has a focus on the effect of introducing reflective practice to a group of Japanese nurses for whom 'reflective practice' was an alien concept. While journals were not specifically mentioned (the term 'workbook' was used), the practice of reflection was written, ongoing and progressive – as in a journal. The challenge to the nurses in respect of the socio-political issues, which they had not previously considered, caused consternation. One said, 'I never thought about these areas before. I was really worried. I was unsure of what I should write down. What were the issues of nursing practices? And what things can I do in order to cope with the issues?' Another commented 'it might be difficult to use reflection in order to cause change because we cannot ignore the physician's authority . . . it is rarely . . . that nurses make decisions for patient care planning without asking doctors'. The study usefully reveals a number of sources of difficulty in introducing journals or reflective practice to groups for whom the questioning in reflective processes does not have a conceptual basis, and such ideas run counter to the general philosophy of the profession or society.

Using journals to support elements of educational programmes

There are a number of examples of journal use that support the particular content of educational programmes. Wetherell and Mullins (1996) describe problem-based learning (PBL) in dentistry, following the example set in medical schools. In this case, journals are used in two areas of a programme to: 'formalize reflection, [provide] an outlet for personal feeling; an opportunity for feedback about a student's progress and about the course; . . . a summary of the year's work; and a means whereby students and teachers gain insight into the learning process.'

One use of journals by Wetherell and Mullins was in an oral diagnosis course that was located in a pain clinic. The course was intended to increase students' responsibility for their learning and self-development. The journal was a vehicle for expression of feelings and to communicate issues of concern to their tutors. Students were asked to write about anxieties and ways in which they felt they could gain more from the clinic experience. The journal content was discussed in one-to-one tutorials. After modifications, around three-quarters of the students favoured the method. Among specific reasons for this, the journal's provision of a record of cases and its value as a 'checklist of things to be learned or done' were cited in particular. These might not have been the most obvious roles for a journal!

Wetherell and Mullins also report on journals used in their first year (PBL) dentistry courses. Students faced four 'streams' and a variety of unfamiliar forms of input. They were given a general introduction to journals as a tool for learning with discussion and a demonstration of existing journals. They were encouraged to explore personal reactions to their experiences. The journals were read by staff and helpful comments were made, but there was no graded assessment. As in many other examples of journal work, reading the journals provided staff with valuable feedback on the curriculum.

In the context of problem-based learning, it is interesting to note comment by Yinger and Clark (1981) about their uses of journals with teachers: 'given the opportunity to write about and reflect on what they were doing, remarkable and exciting changes took place. Much to their surprise, they found themselves solving problems . . . that had previously been wearing them down.'

The development of learning journals within study programmes is rarely a smooth one – and yet the papers that are eventually published usually concern only the final result when the journal work is agreed to be successful. Stephani et al. (2000), who worked with Environmental Studies postgraduate students, describe the evolution process of the journal work – an evolution that took account of the experiences of the students themselves, though did not accede to calls for a traditional form of assessment. Assessment was also an issue for some students on a programme that enabled lay church members to graduate as ministers (Moon,

2004b). A number of the students commented that they did not know what was required and the fact that journals were, at that stage, assessed, put pressure on them. Some commented that they came to the point of understanding that they may not know what they were meant to be doing – but it was up to them to work out the personal value of the journal through their work in the journal. A later comment from one student though, was that (the task) 'was easier in the second year. I didn't know what I was supposed to be doing but I realized that you have to find out for yourself.'

It is worth remembering, in this section on the role of journals in professional education programmes, that the focus of journals is not always is as a reflective adjunct to professional learning. Journals may, for example, be used as a formal collecting point for evidence that they have achieved the required standards for a programme (e.g. Anon., 'Reflective journals of evidence' (nd)). Journals come in all forms, as we have seen. To find out what a journal is or does, the reader needs a clear statement or has to focus deep into the text of its description.

An example of a collaborative multi-professional journal

Another form of use of journals and reflection in development of practice is demonstrated in reports of collaborative projects. Cowan and Westwood (2004) describe situations in which groups of higher education staff have worked together in order to reflect on their own professional development and practices. Alterio (2004) describes a journal that involved a multi-professional group (four higher education lecturers from different disciplines, two occupational therapists with different kinds of work, two nurses and one estate agent) with wide-ranging subject matter. The group that emerged within the context of a larger research project decided to work on a collaborative journal for a year. They chose not to meet face to face and maintained anonymity through pseudonyms. Other than in the written word of the journal, their communication was only with the researcher. The entries could be about anything and in any written format. Some process issues were agreed as a set of ground rules.

Analysis of the journal content after a year indicated that 'entries were diverse in both genre and content. Content ranged from personal reflections through to professional philosophies. Genres covered poetry to prose. Entries ranged from one paragraph to three pages' (Alterio, 2004). Entries stood alone or linked to others, offering 'fresh insights'. Four topics predominated: practice-related learning, professional philosophies, personal learning and growth and reflective practice. There were also five purposes: to connect with the others involved, to pose questions, the discussion of issues, the sharing of learning and capturing of stories. In other words, the learning from the one journal was diverse. The learners made various comments about the process, but saw it as a valuable form of learning and several subsequently intended to institute similar practices in their workplaces, even though anonymity might be difficult to maintain at work. Alterio comments on the emotional learning that occurred and the way in which the journal provided multiple perspectives (Mortiboys, 2002). In effect, it would seem that the journal enabled the reflective processes of the participants to be deepened through working with others.

Thinkpoint

The following extracts are from *A Room of One's Own*, written by Virginia Woolf in 1929 in an essay about the lack of voice of women in fiction. In the first extract, Woolf is in a library and has ordered books in order to research her query.

> Have you noticed how many books are written about women in one year? Have you any notion how many are written by men? Are you aware that you are, perhaps, the most discussed animal in the universe?
>
> (p. 24)

> What could be the reason, then, of this curious disparity . . . Why are women . . . so much more interesting to men than men are to women? A very curious fact it seemed.
>
> (p. 25)

At this point, a large number of books arrived on her desk in front of her – to 'help' her reach an answer to her question. The student – to whom she refers – was seated beside her in the library.

> The student who has been trained at Oxbridge has no doubt some method of shepherding his question past all distractions till it runs into its answer as a sheep runs into its pen . . . But if, unfortunately, one has had no training in a university, the question, far from being shepherded to its pen, flies like a frightened flock hither and thither, helter skelter, pursued by a whole pack of hounds. Professors, school-masters, sociologists, clergymen, novelists, essayists, journalists, men who had no qualification save that they were not women, chased my simple and single question – Why are women poor? – until it became fifty questions; until the fifty questions leapt frantically into mid-stream and were carried away.
>
> (p. 25)

After much entertaining reflection and deliberation, Woolf concluded that a woman

> must have money and a room of her own if she is to write fiction [and] that, as you will see, leaves the great problem of the true nature of woman and the true nature of fiction, unsolved.
>
> (p. 5)

Chapter 8

Learning journals and personal development

Introduction

There are no sharp lines to be drawn between personal and professional development and it is doubtful that one can develop as an adequate professional in the broader sense without parallel personal developments. The idea of personal development in learning journals, however, generates a wealth of approaches and styles beyond the professional development literature. With some thought and creativity, many of the approaches to journals that are included in this chapter can be or are applied to enrich journal-writing in professional and formal education learning.

The range of enthusiastic writing about personal journals in the literature makes difficult the effort to find a logical structure for this chapter which needs to be informative as well as to capture the rich potential of this form of writing. After several perusals of the literature on personal development journals, some headings that roughly covered the field reluctantly emerged to form the basis of the chapter.

Some general issues in personal learning journals

The intention to engage in personal journal-writing is almost certainly far more prevalent than is the sustained practice. It might be interesting to muse on what all the purchasers of blank journal pages of journals might have written – had they actually got started. The start of journals is perhaps most common at New Year and we might guess that the often flat post-Christmas days of early January are those most commonly recorded before the habit tails off. Another start-time for journals is on holiday or when travelling. It was interesting to observe, recently, the sale of blank books labelled 'journal' at airport shops.

While we take in the full range of journal-writing that is not work-related in this chapter, the focus is largely on journals that are written for longer than the first day of a holiday, and with more purpose than the description of events and scenes. The focus is on situations where there is intention to 'move on' personally. The ways of 'moving on' represent the headings of this chapter but as in previous situations in this book, there are overlaps and the original intentions of a writer may change. Personal development journals may be for 'moving on' by way of provision of personal support, an establishment of personal identity, a therapy, an exploration or the widening of experience or awareness, self-organization, the support of creativity, or the development or support of spirituality. Each of these are explored below in the following sections.

We might dwell for a moment on the main topic of this chapter, which is self-development. When applying the notion of reflection in personal development contexts Moon (1999b), suggests that personal development could usefully be seen as functioning in a deficit or non-deficit situation. The deficit mode is represented by situations of counselling or therapy where the aim is to reach a perceived state of normality. The non-deficit mode of self-development is represented by 'growth' or the aim to reach a (perceived) more successful state. Based on Eraut's (1994) work, it was convenient to see personal development as operating in three notional stages – of self-awareness, self-improvement and self-empowerment – the effort to be aware, the effort to go beyond this and improve, and the reaching out for forms of emancipation.

It would seem that some or much personal development occurs through the agency of better emotional management. Chapter 3 indicated the range of ways in which emotions can impinge on the manner in which a person learns or reflects.

Journals for personal support

'Personal support' is a term to cover a range of ideas around what are probably the most usual reasons for using personal journals – for finding direction, for understanding the self, for keeping things in balance. A journal is a place in which the writers can be authentically themselves and can weave their way through the portrayed selves that they feel are seen by others. Bruner's (1990) concept of 'the construction of a longitudinal version of self' seems particularly relevant to journal-writing.

Some have described their journals as a friend or as company, for example, through transitions. Bridges (1980) suggests that a journal can be particularly helpful during experiences such as divorce or career change – particularly in the space between endings and beginnings that he calls the 'neutral zone'. In a similar way, journals can provide the personal space within which to undertake 'rites of passage'. Allied to the notion of 'friend' is the notion of nurturance. Cooper (1991) suggests that 'Writing in a journal is . . . a way to attend to the self, to care for and to feed oneself'. Cooper talks about journals as places for 'dumping anger, guilt or fear instead of dumping it on those we love' (1991: 105). Rainer (1978) talks of 'putting a scream in the diary'. Helpful 'screams' may come in the form of letters written but not sent, large writing written with a heavy pen or heavy scribble. Working on catharsis in Progoff's (1975) Intensive Journal or with Rainer's techniques might be a matter, for example, of writing a dialogue (Chapter 13) with the agency that represents the cause of the anger – be it person or organization (etc.). From long experience, these techniques do work and this would seem to be the experience of Shepherd (2004) who describes an experience:

keeping a journal can be a cathartic experience. I decided to test this . . . in action and wrote something down that had been troubling me for over 20 years and, having subjected it to reflective inquiry, I now feel less troubled about that event . . . I find . . . that subjecting concerns to interrogation is likely to lead to an outcome of positive action. My journal questions help me identify my concern and allow me to interrogate it to determine why it is that I feel and think about the issue in the way that I do.

(Shepherd, 2004)

It would seem that cathartic experiences of journal-writing may work through emotional insight (Chapter 3) – it is as if a form of non-language-based emotional learning occurs. The learner is only able to perceive change or a state of easing of tension – but is not able to explain it.

Some journal-writing appeals to a strength or wisdom that can be availed through the act of writing reflectively. For example, Rainer talks of the 'silver-lining voice' that comes into her writing, giving her advice, and in a somewhat different example Fox (1982) refers to the support that journal-writing gave to a client of his in his attempts to give up smoking. Progoff formalizes the notion of guidance from wisdom in one of the sections of the Intensive Journal in which writers imagine a dialogue with a person or being who is or has been a source of wisdom in their lives.

Writing a journal over a period of time also provides personal support on personal attitudes and behaviour. One of the most useful sections of the Intensive Journal is the 'period log'. The period log is a section for review of a period of life in which there has been a common theme or direction. More than most other journal-writing activities, it provides a sense of perspective, a sense of rhythm and change and sometimes enables the recognition of the repeat of themes in life. It generates a sense of balance in which it is easier to place the peaks and troughs – the 'mountains and molehills' (Rainer, 1978).

Journals for establishing personal identity

The lives of some people are obviously rich. Before the end of their teens they have undergone more socially diverse experiences than others experience in a lifetime. To gather self-esteem enough to rise beyond a narrow and perhaps fragile lifestyle can be difficult for many without these experiences. Progoff's journal was used as part of a programme for a group of unemployed New York people who were training to take on work as nurse's aides, security guards and other such jobs (Kaiser, 1981). Most were new immigrants, they were black and had few opportunities to help themselves. Ninety per cent of them were keeping the journal after six months, and most succeeded in maintaining the posts which they gained or of bettering themselves in other ways. The programme officials attributed much of the success of the programme to the use of the journal and the manner in which it brought them into touch with their inner selves. They came to value themselves and their capacities.

Along the same lines, Hallberg (1987) talks of journals being 'person-making'. He suggests that the use of journals (such as that of Progoff) 'is far more powerful and far-reaching in its effects than is generally recognized . . . [It is] working to change that student's enduring attitudes, values and sense of personal identity' (1987: 289).

Becoming aware of the range of experiences and valuing them builds a sense of identity or personhood. Fox (1982) describes how a client, a 14-year-old who had been in foster care for most of his life, gathered 'fragments of his life' – photos, ticket stubs and so on – in order to 'define himself' and begin to build a self-image. A journal of this sort serves to position an individual in the present, with an understood past and a clearer future. Rainer (1978) talks of 'rereading yourself' by reading through journal entries. She says that: 'the diarist comes to see patterns of experience and personality . . . The patterns are completely individual and deepen the understanding of one's own nature' (1978: 265). Similarly, Cooper (1991) talks of journals as 'a way to tell our own story, a way to learn who we have been, who we are and who we are becoming. We literally become teachers and researchers in our own lives, empowering ourselves in the process' (1991: 98). Empowerment is seen as the 'integration of . . . own needs, values and desires with the often conflicting views of society or the workplace' (Cooper, 1991: 108).

Journals in therapy

In this section we inevitably overlap with the previous section. However, not all uses of journals in therapy are associated with the establishment of personal identity. Fox describes the use of journal-writing to support behaviour changes and shifts in attitude. One client, for example, found it helpful to examine his smoking behaviour in detail and to locate the type of anxiety that was relieved through smoking. He managed subsequently to give up smoking. Another client, with very rigid attitudes and behaviour, took on a more relaxed personality through writing a journal. The subject matter of his writing was initially formal, but he progressed through free writing and 'rambling' and was able to 'turn away from logical, sequentially ordered thinking towards freer contact with experience and feeling'.

Another therapeutic use of journal-writing is rehearsal of future events that evoke fear. By writing about the (future) event, imagining going through it and behaving calmly, and rereading/reliving the material several times, there is likely to be a beneficial effect on behaviour at the time of the event itself. An example of this application might be a driving test. Rainer (1978) describes behaviour rehearsal in a considerably less clinical context of engendering eroticism, where she suggests that the writer should practise in her journal making requests for fulfilment of her sexual desires.

It was in a context of psychotherapy that Progoff developed the structure of the Intensive Journal. He would ask clients to write in a loose-leaf notebook to record the events of their inner lives. Through noticing the pattern of questions that he asked of clients in relation to their writing, he began to formulate the sections that were subsequently the structure of the published version (Progoff, 1975).

Journals for exploring or widening experience or awareness

One of the writers of journals on a programme to prepare her for ministry said:

> The journal makes you more conscious of things – more aware. You think 'that would be useful to put in the journal' and then hold onto it. It 'highlights' things. It helps you to search for themes. It is useful to go back over your practice. You may not understand at first. You might annotate these things to think about ['unpack'] later. There may also be 'pop-up' issues – or issues in the news. The journal makes you notice things that might otherwise slip by.
>
> (Person 'A', quoted in Moon, 2004b)

A large range of journal-writing belongs in this group. It includes the old idea of a commonplace book, which was like a scrapbook of everyday life. It probably includes most travel and holiday journals that are written to accompany the exploration of external physical journeys (Mallon, 1984). In this respect, Fulwiler's (1986) likening of journal entries to snapshots of life is helpful. He suggests that because he writes a journal and may write about what he experiences, he experiences it with greater awareness.

Journals may also accompany an internal mental journey. There are many descriptions of journals of internal mental journeys of exploration in the literature. Creme's (1998) example of death journals is one. Another is the sex journal undertaken by Anderson's (1982) students in the context of a psychology class. The students were asked to keep a journal of their 'observations of sex in the environment, magazines, TV, people's interactions, etc. and [their] reactions to these observations'. Although the context of this exercise was academic, much of the learning that resulted seems to have been personal and over half of the students reported changing their behaviour or lifestyle as a result of the exercise. As they tried to make sense of what they recorded, they often gained insights. One said, 'As I write this, I realize how, for a lot of women, sex and fear are so interrelated. What do men fear? Women fear men.' Along similar lines, we referred above to Rainer's suggestion of the use of journals to explore eroticism and she also mentions the discovery of joy.

Sometimes the exploration of an issue in journals comes not from a direct confrontation with the object, but by treating it metaphorically. Metaphor can be a way of making explicit the personal theories by which we live (Griffiths and Tann, 1992). It may be a matter of applying metaphors to situations in order to make new understanding from them. For example, Cooper (1991) describes a situation in which a woman described herself as like a diaper pin in her family, 'holding the fabric of our lives together and keeping the crap cleaned off'. She says she is ready to pull out the pin: 'But must I hurt my family to pull out and let the fabric of the diaper find new shape and form – while I let the process of reshaping begin?' (1991: 102).

Joanna Field frequently used metaphor in her use of journals as a means of personal exploration of herself and her abilities to paint (Field, 1952; Milner, 1957, 1987). In her 1951 book, Field describes finding the method of free association as a means to uncovering the deeper meanings of her patterns of behaviour. In another book, written a little later, Milner (now using her own name, and a practising psychoanalyst) records, in a similar way, a further personal project of learning to paint (Milner, 1957). In 1987, she returned to the more generalized theme in *Eternity's Sunrise: A Way of Keeping a Diary* (Milner, 1987), now using metaphor as a means of structuring the manner in which she works in her diary. She focuses on the significance of the 'small private moments that came nuzzling into my thoughts, asking for attention' (synopsis). She interprets these 'bead memories' as 'bridges' or points of integration for the different aspects of mental functioning (feeling, reason and imagination), regarding them as having particular importance for the passage of her consciousness.

We began this section with reference to journals that accompany a journey, whether physical or mental. It is worth noting that Progoff's view of the metaphor of journey is different. He considers that there is a flow within our lives and when we begin to tap into it, we flow with it. Kaiser's (1981) interpretation is: 'There is an underground stream of images in all of us . . . When we enter it, we ride where it wants to go.'

Journals for self-organization

To most people in professional or everyday life, a diary or sometimes even a journal means a small book in which to record events in the future as an aide-memoire and an aid to self-organization. One direction in which these have developed is in the 'pocket organizer', which has specially punched paper to ensure that people tied themselves to purchasing expensive packs of paper. On the whole, this form of diary is a means of recording and noting, and not a journal in the sense used in this book. Not very different from this idea, however, are means of working with journals that do facilitate the organization of one's life and which incorporate sections for the development of ideas. These do come into the range of this book because of the reflective integration section of them which is associated with the owner's thought processes. It is possible that the same organizing notebook could have the integrative nature perceived by one person, while another might not recognize its quality. An example of such a journal is given in Chapter 12.

Journals to support creativity

In one sense, all journal-writing is creative. We construct meanings in the act of writing and creativity is part of the nature of reflective writing. We also need to acknowledge that specifically creative thoughts or insights can emerge unexpectedly from writing about anything. The skill then may be in the recognition of the value of these thoughts. This section deals with journal work and writing that has a particular aim of generating creative ideas – and not all creativity needs to be verbal.

Sometimes a whole journal is devoted towards support or generation of creative ideas. Milner's (1957) description of learning to paint is a powerful example and it is both to its credit and its loss that it is so closely tied to psychoanalytical theory. Alternatively the search for creativity may be focused in specific journal activities. A number of activities with this function are described in Chapter 13. One that seems particularly relevant is the 'dialogue with works' (Progoff, 1975) in which a written dialogue is held with a proposed or ongoing project. It is a way of focusing on the intrinsic qualities of the project or 'work' and of avoiding the pressure of rationality or the influence or habit of others.

There seem to be a number of ways in which journal-writing might enhance creativity. Miller (1979) suggests that the act of writing may generate creative ideas but also that 'writing the immediate thoughts makes more "room" for new avenues of thinking'. She suggests that writing allows the mind to 'explore more freely since we do not run the risk of losing our previous thoughts'. This may indicate why a project journal can come to feel so important (Chapter 12).

Working with dreams is a different means of generating ideas that are unexpected, but this inconveniently depends on the somewhat unpredictable process of dreaming and remembering dreams (Shohet, 1985). For some, Progoff's techniques of reaching 'twilight' states are a more reliable means of accessing sources of 'the unexpected'. 'Twilight imagery' is a state in which one is deeply relaxed and has attention 'turned inwards'. Images begin to arise and they are recorded. The very act of recording and valuing the images seems to induce more images. Work in this mode 'feels' highly creative, but it may or may not have an obvious application to any particular current issue.

Writing a journal may also capture ideas for creative activities or as memories like the notebook that is graphically described by Didion (1968):

> I sometimes delude myself about why I keep a notebook, imagine that some thrifty virtue derives from preserving everything observed. See enough and write it down, I tell myself, and then, some morning when the world seems drained of wonder . . . – on that bankrupt morning, I will simply open my notebook and there it will all be, a forgotten account with accumulated interest, paid passage to the world out there.
>
> (Didion, 1968: 115, 116)

Journals in the development or exploration of spirituality

Journal-writing can be an important activity in the development of both secular and religious spirituality. We have described in other chapters Walker's use of journals with potential leaders in a religious community (Walker, 1985) and it is interesting to note the wide use of Progoff's Intensive Journal in religious communities. Elements of the work with the Intensive Journal particularly lend themselves to spiritual exploration both in the depth of working and the structures of the exercises. Indeed the manner in which Progoff describes the Intensive Journal could be said to generate a sense of depth, an air of mystique or reverence – that is well borne out in the atmosphere of an Intensive Journal workshop.

We have also quoted from journals that were used in a programme for the development of lay people towards the ministry (Moon, 2004b). Some of the comments of participants illustrate the role that journals had in their development. Person C said 'I wanted a "joined-up" approach to (this) training – to link secular and church work and the journal enabled this. This holistic approach to training and developing me as a person was very helpful. I can carry on this type of process now I am ordained. It is a joined-up approach'. Another (Person F) commented that she had not found the journal process easy at first, partly because of the theological processes. Though she had been a lifelong Christian, the experience had not been one of questioning and thinking about issues or of enlarging knowledge, but of accepting and the journal encouraged the development of her critical views. She also said that she had engaged in a previous theology course and it was the journal in this course that had enabled her to pull together the previous experiences.

In a somewhat similar form of spirituality, Wolf Moondance (1994) describes the use of spirit journals to provide a record of feelings and a place for the recording of dreams in the learning of native American spirit medicine. She describes ways of deepening the sense of ownership of the journal with pictures, beads and sequins. She suggests that the material of dreams, memories and other recording should be written in paragraphs, not half-sentences, because 'you'll need to make sense of what is being said to you' by 'the inner self . . . in the spirit world' (1994: 21). The entries should be dated, with the time noted and a brief reference to the place in which the writing is done ('a little bit about what is going on around you' (1994: 21)). She talks of the need to revere the journal, taking care of it and carrying it – 'Your respect for the journal is very important. It teaches you respect for yourself' (1994: 21). Interestingly, the sense of powerful ownership, of deep personal valuing of the writing process in a journal that these words portray, is no stranger to other keepers of personal journals. They do feel bound up intimately with 'myself' (Shepherd, 2004).

Thinkpoint

Alan Bennett tells of his childhood thoughts just after his father's death.

> A few weeks after he dies I go to Scotland . . . it is early evening when I arrive and so I sit . . . in the last of the sunshine and make some notes about my father.
>
> He always washed up . . .
>
> He always wore black shoes.
>
> He often picked up stuff in the street – coins, naturally, but which pleased him out of all proportion to their value; nuts, screws, bits that had fallen off cars. Mam disapproved of this habit lest things might be dirty.
>
> He had no smell at all and . . . scarcely a grey hair, paleish blue eyes and a worn red face brimming over with kindness and pleasure. When he washed, he dried his face so vigorously that it squeaked.
>
> (Bennett, A., 2000: 47)

Chapter 9

Starting to write a learning journal

Introduction

For some, writing reflectively in a journal is no problem. They take to it like the proverbial duck takes to her water. Some, however, struggle (Dart *et al.*, 1998). They want more structure or writing in this way feels unfamiliar; it may feel 'wrong' because their training since school has been to write more formally, not, for example, using the first person. The demise of letter writing may have something to do with the difficulty because a letter to a friend can be similar to a journal entry in style and experience of writing. We do, on the other hand, use email.

Not only may learners have difficulty with journal-writing, but, similarly, so may their teaching staff. There is no reason why most higher education staff should automatically know how to write reflectively in a sustained manner. Those who have encountered formal education themselves more recently, however, may have been asked to engage in some forms of reflective practice.

Beyond this introductory section, this chapter considers, from several angles, how to start to write a learning journal. We look at issues in the management of journal-writing, at ways of presenting the task of journal-writing and of getting learners started. We also look at ways of improving writing and at some of the difficulties that may be encountered. The chapter provides a basis for those who might plan to use or to introduce journal-writing, or for those who might want to start a journal for themselves.

The management of journal-writing (mainly in the context of formal education)

In the preparation of this book, a number of situations have become evident where journals have been introduced without much **forethought**. The use of a learning journal 'just seemed like a good idea'. Such thinking has often come about under the pressure to institute personal development planning in higher education. Good preparation however, may mean that the exercise is sustained, with a more substantial and satisfying outcome in terms of learning. However, while forethought is important, it is unlikely that a journal will be 'right' initially. Journal-writing evolves with the experiences of the learners and the teaching staff (Ashbury *et al.*, 1993).

A first consideration in setting up a journal is the **purpose** of the task. Chapter 5 reviewed many purposes for which journals have been used, or that they have fulfilled. Being clear as to why a journal task is set lays the basis for planning, for inducting learners into the task, for the structure (if any) of the journal and for assessment. The aim needs to be made clear to anyone concerned in the project. The aim and the intended journal task also need to **fit within course design**. Creme (1998) indicates that the **level of integration** of a journal task within a programme is also likely to be an influence on its success. The purpose may be 'driven' by PDP initiatives, or by the nature of the programme itself. In the latter case, the use of a journal will need to be directed towards meeting the statements of learning outcome (Moon, 2002).

One manner of hinting at the purpose of a journal is represented in the *title* that is given to a journal. We discussed some of the terms used to describe learning journals in Chapter 1. The title may generally indicate the type of activity involved in keeping the journal, such as in Creme's three examples of a 'project journal', a 'record of study' and the 'death journal'.

The management of journal-writing involves anticipation of the tasks involved and the demands that may arise from it. **Managing the demands** from a small class is very different from managing the demands from a large class with over 50 students and there are some recommendations that might be considered in the literature that the journals are best suited to small groups of learners who are relatively mature (Stephani, 1997; Hettich, 1990). On the other hand, there are plenty of examples of the relatively sophisticated use of journals in larger classes, and with young children (e.g. Mayher *et al.*, 1983). A significant variable in management of journals is the degree of **monitoring and assessment** that are planned. Reading journals may be more enjoyable than reading essays (November, 1993) but it can take a long time, particularly if feedback is required to be written. One method of time-saving on feedback is the use of an audiotape.

A reason why journal-writing may, in some ways, be easier with young children is because **trust** and assessment may be less sensitive issues. Journal-writing will work best in an atmosphere of trust (Mayher *et al.*, 1983). If the environment is not supportive, it is likely to be the environment that becomes the topic of journal-writing. Older students, who are aware of the potential consequences of assessment, need assurance that there is relaxation of concern for the usual elements of writing that matter, such as spelling, construction, and use of formal language. But there will be concerns about the manner in which journals will be monitored or assessed, particularly among students who are not even sure on what they are expected to write however many times this may have been explained (Francis, 1995).

Trust is an issue also for staff. By setting up an **openness in the learning situation**, Wetherell and Mullins (1996) suggest that they expose themselves to criticism in students' journals. They cannot be defensive, or take offence because they have invited the open atmosphere. They must deal with student criticism, which may be misdirected or unfounded, without aggravating the situation, and in away that leads to a positive resolution.

Trust between staff and students is also important because journal-writing can generate unexpected emotions. Such writing can 'pose a threat to the writer by revealing what lies beneath carefully constructed defenses' (Mayher *et al.*, 1983: 34). Similarly, writing can initiate dramatic changes in a learner's life patterns (Moon, 1999b). There are, for example, stories of students who leave courses after they have the opportunity to explore their feelings in a journal (e.g. Cooper, 1991). This event may be positive for the individual, but it involves considerable management skills on the part of staff.

Clearly the issue of assessment relates to the trust atmosphere. If learners are required to write journals that are not judged by another, the trust issue is different from situations in which journals are overseen by staff, and different again from those in which journals are graded. Where journals are read, the issues of **privacy or confidentiality** emerge and, to some extent, the more that the learners trust the staff member, the more they are likely to feel comfortable about revealing.

Where journals are used for **assessment** (see Chapter 10) and where the marks are significant, not only is the openness of the writer potentially under greater threat but they may write according to what they think the assessor wants. We have described the example of students who decided that 'self-flagellation' was what their tutors wanted to read about (Salisbury, 1994). Staff, may vary in their sympathy for and comprehension of the task of journal-writing (Salisbury, 1994). It is not unlikely that students writing a journal for the same purpose may receive very different qualities of feedback from different members of staff overseeing or even marking equivalent work. Mayher *et al.* (1983) advise teachers who are overseeing journals: '. . . be relaxed. Don't overwhelm students with the task, but allow it to develop organically, letting it work for them in ways they discover. By encouraging and gently prodding . . . journal-writing can open up new learning channels in your curriculum' (1983: 25).

Time is an issue in journal-writing for staff and learners. Journal-writing creates an intellectual space for learners, but equally, it is the time that it takes that is a major reason for the abandonment of journal-writing. The time issue needs to be managed. Some apparently successful journals arise from regular opportunities to write either at the beginning or at the end of classes, sometimes responding to the class content (e.g. Hahnemann, 1986). However, it is possible that the classroom is not the place that is most conducive to reflection and some teaching staff would argue that they need all of the time available for teaching (and not, they thereby seem to suggest, for helping students to learn!).

Time, of course, relates to the cost–benefit sum. While there are some reports of the **evaluation** of journal-writing in the literature, it is probable that the analysis of the benefits for students against the 'cost' in terms of time, staff and student effort is mostly a 'gut feeling'. A problem with any evaluation process is how to choose the criteria against which to evaluate the exercise, and this takes us, in classroom situations, back to purpose, learning outcomes, programme design and assessment.

Ethical issues in journal-writing

Ethical issues in journal-writing can seem to make the use of journals too difficult to manage. This is a shame – and an issue that could be taken to the roots of the act of education. Ethical issues are important and, in sensitive situations, they need to be discussed among staff and with learners. In this section we review some of the ethical issues that are involved in journal use (but not assessment – see Chapter 10).

We start by taking **a broad view of the potential ethics of a journal task**. We need to acknowledge several things. First, in ethical concerns, journals are not to be completely separated from other work that students submit. Placement reports can generate just as sensitive a set of issues as a journal. Those who are themselves uncomfortable about reflection may use ethical concerns to bar the way of journal use. Second, a journal task that does not go outside the learner's hands – and which is not assessed, is much freer from potential ethical issues than those that are see by others (i.e. teachers or other learners) – but it may not be written! If journal activity is seen to be of value to the learner's learning, and the student will not engage in it unless it is seen or assessed, then seeing or assessing it can be justified. An ethical issue that can arise even where journals are not seen concerns students who seem to write themselves into states of depression or despair. It is unlikely that the despair has come from 'nowhere', but journal-writing may 'spark it off' – as might other events. Teachers who manage journal activities need to be able to talk to each other about concerns about individual students and need to know where their limits as teachers are, and how to refer to appropriate others. Fenwick (2001) points out that the teacher who becomes concerned about the vulnerability expressed by a student has a difficult dilemma in deciding whether or not to take action. If she approaches the student about what has been written, she moves into a therapeutic kind of relationship with the student – which is significantly different from that of the teacher in its implications for interaction.

The level of **self-disclosure** that is appropriate in professional development journals is a difficult matter on which to guide students and on which to make judgements in assessment. Guidance needs to take account of the cultural background of the students (Stockhausen and Kawashima, 2002; Rothwell and Ghelipter, 2003). While it is appropriate to discuss this matter with students with regard to the use of journals, the regulation of personal and professional issues is a capacity that all such students need to learn. Journals bring this matter to the fore, sometimes in uncomfortable ways from which students need to learn. They do, however, have to learn the lessons from somewhere. Such discomfort is not a good reason to abandon journal-writing.

Another general issue is '**honesty**'. The word is in inverted commas because it is contentious. In setting up a journal that is to be seen or assessed, we have to recognize that what is written by the learner is likely to be modified to relate to the perceived view of those who would see it. This is acknowledged in the development of two definitions for reflective learning (Chapter 1) and our references to Salisbury's self-flagellating sample. It is not acknowledged in a statement such as 'To be effective in promoting learning, journal-writing necessitates that students be honest and open in their entries' (Thorpe, 2004). What is honesty? When Jaye (2001) wrote accounts of an emotionally upsetting influence in her life on subsequent occasions after the event, the accounts differed. The exercises provided in the resources section (Resources 3, 4 and 5) illustrate the same point. Asking students to write about an emotional event in the manner described above is helpful to them in their general understanding of journal work. There is not necessarily one truth about an event and this is a fundamental point of understanding that needs to be present for the teachers involved in journal work. Understanding the idea of truth and uncertainty in knowledge is developmental and learners will come to that understanding through maturation and through work such as the use of journals (Baxter Magolda, 1992; King and Kitchener, 1994; Moon, 2004a).

Ethical issues should be viewed in relation to the **purpose** for which a journal is used and the purpose should take account of ethical issues, as well as those in the preceding paragraph. If the purpose of the journal is to enhance reflective practice in a professional setting – then the student needs to be addressing the ethical issues in the content and process of writing a journal. If the purpose is to enhance creativity – then there may be some issues in the process, but ethics as a topic may not come into the content.

A fear of some who manage journals is that **material of a sensitive nature might be revealed** (English, 2001). We have already mentioned students who reveal personal vulnerabilities above. Students have been known to reveal their role in criminal activity. This potentially places the reader of such a journal in the position of accessory after the crime – with many implications. Another area of sensitivity may arise in a placement, where the learner, in being critically reflective discusses shortcomings that she perceives in named staff or activities of an organization. Sometimes students in placements such as hospitals or legal situations are party to case notes and can carelessly or naively reveal confidential information. The potential that issues such as those described in this paragraph might arise should be anticipated as much as possible in the setting up of the journal and, in the context of a broad discussion of confidentiality, learners need to be helped to see what is and is not appropriate. Examples may help. English provides a number of case studies to illustrate her discussion of the general teaching issues, but there is good reason to use examples to illustrate the matter with learners – for most, the ethical education that this entails will also be relevant to their studies.

A discussion of confidentiality needs to take into consideration the identity of those who might view a journal. Building in some peer review of journals, or joint reflection is often very beneficial to the reflective learning in providing different perspectives, but what might it do to confidentiality issues? If the journal is to be seen by a teacher, is it just one tutor? If a tutor has doubts, can she show it to another tutor or a more senior teacher? Furthermore, what about **external examiners or external moderation processes**? Rothwell and Ghelipter (2003) illustrate this point in relation to the Israeli students with whom they worked. Some of the students were employed in military services or security forces and they specifically requested that their journals should not be in the external moderation sample – but such a request generates other ethical issues about fairness in teaching . . .

Presenting the task of writing a journal

This section looks at how to guide the students, what to tell them, how to help them to start their writing. The development of the ability to write reflectively is the subject matter of the last section in this chapter.

The medium for journals

Journals do not need to be on paper and hence an early decision is on the medium for recording. There are advantages and disadvantages to every medium. Electronic journals, are very easy to communicate to another who has compatible equipment – but they are not as portable as paper and pen. An intermediate method is to word-process a journal, but to present it on paper. There is some evidence that writing on a computer has different qualities from those of writing in hand (Bunker and Cronin, 1997) – but the qualities may not be the wrong ones. Recording on audiotape is quick, but it is less easy to 'flick though' or review and there are suggestions that it tends to consist more of descriptive than reflective work (Ficher, 1990). Video could also have possibilities. With the common use of digital photography, particularly on mobile phones, graphic journals are possible, too – or the mixing of written and graphic work.

Format and form

Unless there are reasons for prescribing a particular format, it is desirable that the format of a journal is a matter for personal experiment and choice for the learner because this is a manner through which a sense of ownership – a relationship to the writing – is developed. Rainer (1978) points out how the 'rigid design of those one- and five-year' calendar styles of diary influence the manner of writing. There is a specific space to fill and pages of emptiness ahead'. There is advantage in an unstructured format, and, from the point of view of flexibility, even more advantage in using loose-leaf arrangements. Loose leaves can be written independently from the journal itself and added, enhancing portability. Leaves, however, can also be torn out! Size of the journal may be an issue. Rainer suggests that small books may produce a 'compressed writing style', while they have obvious advantages for portability (Grumet, 1990). A flimsily covered journal has no chance of lasting for long. With a hard cover, the journal will last and the cover frees the writer from the need to seek other surfaces for support when writing. The format of a journal may be required to provide space for feedback or contributions from another. Wagenaar (1984) asks his students to leave one sheet of each double entry blank for the comments of tutors.

General instructions on writing a journal

There are instructions that are either helpful or essential when a journal task is first given. Most of them require some decision making in advance and many can be given on a sheet of 'guidelines'. Several writers provide useful lists of instructions (e.g. Walker, 1985; Fulwiler, 1986; Salisbury, 1994). Matters to do with the technique of writing reflectively are dealt with in the next section.

The purpose of the journal and the explanation of why the journal task is being set

Journals, as a writing task are often 'just given' as part of a programme. After a year or two of use, they become part of the 'wallpaper' – just like lectures, seminars and essays. More than the other structures of a programme, it is important to tell students why they are being asked to write, what they might expect to get out of the experience and how the purpose relates to the format, design, guidelines and, in particular, any assessment tasks. It is particularly useful to give examples. Coltrinari and Mitchell (1999) describe giving instructions and details of a professional journal in a series of four videos.

For more mature learners, it may be useful to provide some theory about the way in which journal-writing might enhance their learning or professional development. Journal-writing is often used, for example, to enhance reflection in practice. It is helpful for the journal to be introduced alongside this theory and it may be appropriate to talk about the way in which journal-writing can support deep learning. Another area of theory with which it is appropriate to introduce journal-writing is that of the social construction of knowledge (Cell, 1984; Ross, 1989; Grumet, 1990). Learners can then see their work in journals as a form of building personal theory.

There are a number of reports in the literature that indicate that students may find the step from formal academic writing to the personalized writing that is characteristic of journals to be problematic. They may need to be told several times, and possibly guided by feedback as to the kind of writing that is desirable in a journal – or more often, what journal-writing is generally not appropriate. November (1993) talks of how he needs to wean his students from 'finished productitis' – the need to tidy and conclude writing in the way in which it is required in an essay. They need to learn that spelling, style, grammar and completion are not necessarily a part of the process of good journal-writing. They may also need to be helped with the idea of using the first person ('I'). Greenhalgh and Hurwitz (1998) and, in particular, Gelter (2003) provide some useful ideas on this. The latter talks of the 'evolutionarily recent "I"' – and of the change of consciousness from 'me' to 'I'. 'Reflection . . . is an important ethical tool to take control of your life, letting the conscious 'I' use social and personal values to guide your actions rather than simple survival values determined by the 'me', which can easily be controlled by others'.

Whether the journal is voluntary or compulsory

Learners may be more willing to work on a journal that is 'strongly advised' or 'will enhance your learning', rather than one that is mandatory . . . or they may not do it at all. An important question is how and where the learning journal fits into the learner's programme of study and the relevant learning outcomes.

Assessment

The decision to assess or not assess journals is discussed in Chapter 10. If journals are to be assessed, it is fair to learners to tell them in advance how they are to be assessed and to consider the assessment criteria on which the process will be based. Assessing journals can be time-consuming. One possibility is to mark a certain number of pages or sections only, and to ask learners to decide which those parts should be. Learners could mark them with yellow sticky notes. They may also need to number pages to facilitate this.

Separate from assessment, there may be **other arrangements for monitoring and providing feedback on journals** – (see also Chapter 10). The frequency for reviewing the progress of learners will depend on many variables, including the nature of the feedback that is to be given. Sometimes the learner may be expected to respond to the tutor's comment and a form of dialogue is developed. As a generalization, most journals used with tertiary students seem to be viewed once or twice a semester. However, Wagenaar (1984) comments that viewing three times a term is necessary for appropriate provision of feedback. It may be helpful to students to take in their journals more frequently in the early days in order to give them guidance and feedback. The comments made by a tutor may be a useful subject matter for the later entries (Gibbs, 1988).

We have discussed confidentiality earlier in the chapter with reference to ethical issues. It is important as an issue in the management of journal-writing and as information for learners. The need for considerations about confidentiality will depend on the purpose of the journal and the sort of material that a learner is likely to write. However, it could be argued that for a journal to impinge significantly on a learner's processes, the exploration of personal and possibly sensitive material is valuable. Monitoring or an assessment process may dissuade a student from engaging at this level. One means of overcoming this problem is to allow learners to tape together pages that they do not wish to be read – or to use a loose-leaf format.

Learners may be invited formally or informally to **read or share their journals with peers**. Sharing material can encourage the writers themselves through comments made, but also can also inspire others in the range and depth of their writing. Sharing may be in pre-arranged sessions, but experience suggests that the option to read material to another, as opposed to paraphrasing it, should be a decision for the student. There are some ways of instituting peer support described in Chapter 13.

Chapter 5 introduced a range of possible structures for journals. Structure can be a means of helping learners to start writing as well as a means to ensure that their reflection 'moves on'. It is not unusual for structures to be suggested but not mandatory – or learners maybe asked to start with a given structure and then to design a structure of journal that suits them.

Structures may not emanate from the journal, but may arise as a consequence of the manner in which a journal task is set. For example, Hahnemann (1986) describes how her (nursing) students are asked to write in their journals at the beginning of a class for around ten minutes. There are also pauses during lectures for writing. Brief assignments are given such as 'write for five minutes on what you have learned about group processes'. The students are also given topics for brief reflection at home.

The material content of a journal

We have tended to consider the content of a journal as writing but depending on the purpose for a journal, other material may be appropriate. There is, for example, no clear division between journals and portfolios where much other material may be presented and linked by reflective writing. Learners may be asked to include academic papers or newspaper articles on which they are asked to reflect. Drawings or photographs or other graphic material may take a principal role in some journals – or a supporting role in others. Wagenaar's sociology students added cartoons or comic strips to illustrate points that they wished to make (Wagenaar, 1984).

It is worth remembering that there are different forms of writing and the use of a variety of forms can greatly enhance the benefits of journals. Poetry, lists, concept maps and other forms interrogate the writer's capacity in different ways that enhance learning.

The length of a journal or the entries in it

Length is not a measure of the quality of the learning that might result from writing a journal. Very brief writing, that does no more than fulfil the minimum require-ments, probably results in little learning. Few seem to give indications of how much learners should write. There are several comments, however, on the varia-tion in the amount that is written. Burnard (1988) talks about receiving both full A4-size binders and a few pages for similar journal tasks from the same group.

The frequency of writing entries

This probably requires guidance. The instruction to write weekly seems to be common (e.g. Ghaye and Lillyman, 1997; Burnard, 1988), though Morrison (1990) suggests a minimum limit of twice a term. He also advises students not to try to write up their journals 'at the last moment' before they are handed in. The instruction on the frequency of writing may be modified by suggestions that students keep more regular notes in a notebook to facilitate their writing. Alternatively there might be instructions to learners to reread their entries regularly and to make further comments as a result (e.g. Ghaye and Lillyman, 1997).

The 'when' and 'where' of writing a journal

This is likely to be dictated by the nature of the task set. It is worth noting, however, that the format of a journal can dictate when and where it is written more than any other factor. The possibility of writing in a handbag- or pocket-sized journal makes the activity more flexible than the use of essentially a non-transportable journal. The ability to write at any time can be liberating. Palm-top computers can be an aid to mobility.

Sometimes it is worth thinking about the **audience** in writing a journal. Gibbs' students, who wrote comments about journal-writing, considered that identification of an audience may 'allow you to give direction to your thinking' (Gibbs, 1988: 99). The writing may not be for the self. Even if the other 'audience' does not, in reality, see the journal, the sense of audience will influence the manner of writing. Elbow and Clarke make this point strongly: 'An audience is a field of force. The closer we come, the more we think about these readers – the stronger the pull they exert over the contents of our minds' (1987: 19). The audience may be the tutor, peers, a grandchild (Rainer, 1978), a mentor or an imaginary figure. Holly (1991) comments that when she writes material for others, 'I am more able to speak clearly (and concisely) to the topic'. If the 'audience' is, indeed, self, then it is worth thinking about which self – the self now or the self in the future – when the journal might be reread.

Writing reflectively

There are two issues in helping students to write reflectively in learning journals. We have noted that many learners are not sure how to write reflectively at all and the first stage is to help them to get started in their reflective writing. However, as we have noted in the discussion of depth and quality in reflective writing, it is difficult to get students to write other than superficially and in a descriptive manner which might seem to reduce the quality of the potential learning (Betts, 2004; Rothwell and Ghelipter, 2003). Moon (2004a) used these two observations of students as the basis of a structure that was designed to facilitate the development of good quality reflective writing and reflective learning ('A two-stage approach to introducing reflective activities'). The generic framework for reflective writing (Chapter 4) also provides an underpinning to the design of the stages. The first of the two stages is termed 'Presenting reflection'. A model – which is reproduced in Figure 9.1 below – guides the kinds of activities that are appropriate for this stage, and in the subsequent pages there are exercises that support the learning in each of the ways depicted in the model (Moon, 2004a).

The other stage of the two-stage model is that of facilitating deeper reflection. Again the model is presented (see Figure 9.2) and again, in Moon 2004a, there can be found a number of exercises following the model.

It is suggested that the students are given some of the exercises from 'Presenting reflection' so that they can begin to write reflectively. Once they are reasonably competent, the exercises from 'facilitating deeper reflection' can be given.

In this book there are three examples from the exercises that are detailed in Moon (2004a) (in Resources 3–5), the instructions for using the exercises (Resource 1) and the generic framework for reflective writing (Resource 2). The development of the exercises is described in Chapter 4 and they can be used at both of the stages that are mentioned above. With three examples in this book and a further three in the other book, it is possible to run the same exercises several times, initially to get learners started with reflection, and later to enable them to deepen their reflective activity. When they are being used to get students started with reflection (the first stage), it may better, with the four-part exercises, to only use the first three parts.

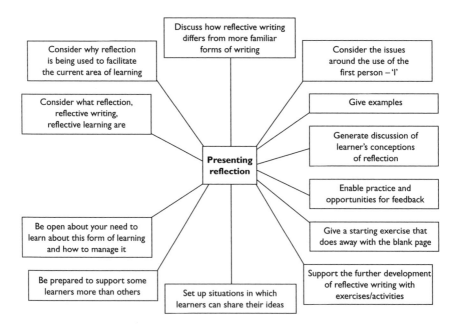

Figure 9.1 Presenting reflection.

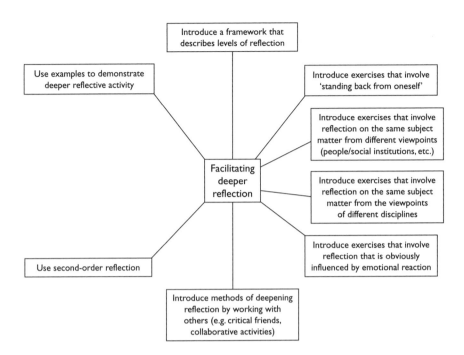

Figure 9.2 Facilitating deeper reflection.

Other ways of getting started with a journal

There are many resources for the development of reflective writing in Moon (2004a).

Some consider that free writing techniques are a valuable means of starting. The writers are encouraged simply to write for a certain length of time – whatever comes into their minds, feelings, thoughts, observations, anything (Rainer, 1978). The results are probably best treated as an exercise increasing the flow of writing, though free writing may be developed as part of a longer exercise (Yinger and Clark, 1981).

Questions are widely used as a means of starting journal writers. It is much easier to answer a question than to generate new material. Questions may guide the journal writer's sequence of thinking (Carlsmith, 1994), and Johns (1994) developed a set of questions for nurse education which focus on reactions to and actions following from an event that has occurred. Morrison (1990, 1996) developed several sets of questions to aid the reflective processes of teacher education students. The questions guide the process of journal-writing so that initially there is a focus on describing, then on organizing and reviewing the material and finally on analysis of, and reflection on, the material. Others have used theoretical constructs such as the Kolb cycle of experiential learning or questionnaires on learning styles. There are also several descriptions of the use of autobiographical tasks as a starting point for journals (e.g. Knowles, 1993; November, 1993). Bolton and Styles (1995) give a useful account of an autobiography workshop.

It seems particularly helpful to show students examples of well-constructed journals, perhaps from previous students (e.g. Redwine, 1989). Wagenaar (1984) suggests that examples of good journals are put on reserve in a library together with comments from the tutor. An alternative to this is to ask students at the end of the year to write advice to students who will be starting journals in the following year, such as descriptions by Walker (1985) and Gibbs (1988). The engineering students described by Gibbs did this by brainstorming on ideas for advice. They shared out the ideas for a writing-up stage and then circulated the notes for comment. The advice was then made available for other students. The advice given in these two papers is addressed to the learners and it includes the following:

• *Make the journal your own*   The journal is 'an extension of yourself, not something outside of you', its usefulness 'can be in proportion to the extent to which it is your own' (Walker, 1985: 54).

• *Be honest*   'Be frank and honest in your entries' (Walker, 1985: 55).
   'You can only learn from your journal if you have enough courage to face yourself as you really are' (Gibbs, 1988: 99).

• *Let words flow*   'Write about whatever is at the top of your mind' (Gibbs, 1988: 98).
   'Get down to it . . . write, write, write . . . let it flow, uncensored and in whatever order it comes. It is very useful simply to write and then to reflect on what has been written' (Walker, 1985: 55).
   'Once you have got going, ideas will tend to lead on to other ideas and before you know it, you will be into your journal' (Gibbs, 1988: 98).

• *Use your own words*   Be informal, use simple English that makes you realize exactly what you meant when you review your journal' (Gibbs, 1988: 98).
   'Use your own words, put your own name on things. Say what you feel, and if that makes you feel guilty, record that and work with it further' (Walker, 1985: 55).

• *Dig deeper*   'Urge yourself to keep digging deeper and deeper so that you can understand and use your understanding. Try to work towards "truths" you have discovered through your experiences; [towards] advice to yourself about what to do in the near future; [and towards] finding questions that you need to think about next, about issues which you don't yet fully understand but need to understand' (Gibbs, 1988: 100).

• *Be flexible* 'Do not be rigid in the way you keep [the journal] . . . Be prepared to try different methods, so that you can mould this exercise to your personal talents and needs' (Walker, 1985: 55).

• *Write things up as soon as you can* 'There is a very definite advantage in being able to record things as quickly as possible, even though one may not immediately write them up fully' (Walker, 1985: 55).

• *Seek help if necessary* 'Feel free to seek help . . . from others: fellow participants, or other people who have used this type of exercise, or the facilitators of the programme' (Walker, 1985: 56).

• *Be selective* Walker (1985: 56) suggests that most of the participants recognized that in the beginning they wrote a great deal more than was necessary. 'Selectivity was a sign of experience.'

Ways of improving work on journals

Here we go beyond the start of learning journal-writing. The methods presented in this section fall into three groups. The first group involves developments in the journal as a physical entity. The second group consists of methods that encourage students to overview their writing (secondary reflection/taking a meta-view). The third involves other mechanisms to deepen the learning from a journal.

Improving the organization of learning journals

There are various reasons why journal writers might want to think of new ways of organizing their journals. They may be required to refer to it within an essay, for example, and we have suggested above that some, but not all of a journal may be marked or assessed by a teacher, with the choice of which parts are to be marked left to the learner. Both of these examples might indicate that the pages of a journal maybe numbered, and, perhaps, the contents listed. It might be appropriate to divide writing into sections – structuring the journal like a double entry journal, for example. Progoff's Intensive Journal provides ideas for many other sections (Chapter 12).

Other methods of organizing journal-writing – perhaps one could say 'making the journal work better for you' – involve emphasizing, making headings, high-lighting and marking in cross references. Cross-references might be identified by symbols, icons, colour, stickers, coloured paper and so on. The use of different pens or different colours can enable a different form of self-expression. Holly (1991) comments that sometimes 'red "feels" right; at other times it's green'. She suggests also that comments might be made in the margin in different colours at a later reread. It is possible to underline or circle (Walker, 1985), to use arrows and asterisks and even to cut and paste (Voss, 1988). Allied to these forms of marking might be techniques, suggested by Progoff (1975), of summarizing periods of time or events in a single image.

Taking a meta-view of learning journal work

The work of Hettich, described above, also provides an example of the fourth group of methods of improving writing in learning from journals. It involves a metacognitive approach. Chapter 3 indicates reasonable evidence that a means by which journals improve learning is through their enhancement of metacognition, that is, taking an overview of one's learning processes. This can be exploited in journals by:

- focusing the attention of learners on to their processes of learning as part of the work that they do in the journal;
- like Hettich (1990), above, by asking them to analyse aspects of their entries for qualities of learning (e.g. by use of Bloom's taxonomy);
- asking them to review the whole process of keeping a journal in relation to the learning that results from it. There are a number of reports of evaluation of journals (e.g. Hahnemann, 1986; Wetherell and Mullins, 1996; Ghaye and Lillyman, 1997), but none seem to be focused directly on the intention to improve learning from subsequent journal or reflective writing.

A variation on these methods of meta-viewing of journals, which fits also in the second section on facilitation, is the situation in which staff choose to write journals alongside their students (e.g. Knowles, 1993; Miller, 1983) and to share entries, particularly those on the processes of journal-writing.

Deepening learning

This book has provided a set of exercises to enable learners to understand the nature of deeper qualities of reflective learning – the basic framework for reflective writing (Resource 2) a number of exercises that are based on the framework (Resources 3, 4, 5) and instructions for the use of these exercises (Resource 1). The background of the development of this material is described in Chapter 4 These should enable learners to deepen their reflective writing because it will enable them better to understand what it is that they are required to do.

There are other methods of helping students to deepen the quality of their learning in journals. These may involve work alone or with colleagues (e.g. the use of 'critical friends' (Sagor, 1991; Francis, 1995) – see Chapter 13. There are a number of theoretical frameworks that may be helpful (e.g. Bloom's taxonomy, Bloom, 1956 – see also Joyce (nd), Perry (1970) and Belenky *et al.* (1986) – used by Hettich (1990), King and Kitchener (1994).

Difficulties that may be encountered in journal-writing

We have said several times before in several contexts that some learners have difficulty in writing reflectively or in a journal. However, it is possible that those who have the most difficulty in the beginning stand to be those who can gain the most from the exercise (Handley, 1998).

The literature provides a range of reasons why learners might find journal-writing difficult. For example: some learners resist, not seeing the relevance of journal-writing to their current pursuit (Francis, 1995; Hatton and Smith, 1995); some are cynical or feel that 'reflection' is overemphasized (James and Denley, 1993; Salisbury, 1994) or concerned that they will not produce what the teacher wants, or they are too concerned to produce what they perceive to be wanted (Dillon, 1983). Many are reported to request more guidance or structure (Ashbury *et al.*, 1993; Heath, 1998; Dart *et al.*, 1998). Students on courses often feel that they do not have time to engage in an activity whose value may not be as obvious at the time (Hettich, 1976; Francis, 1995). They are likely, perhaps misguidedly, to assume that they learn more from traditional approaches to teaching because they are traditional.

These are just some of the reasons cited by students for procrastination. Many students have study habits that do not accord with regular journal entries in that they let tasks accumulate and only under pressure make the due effort (Canning, 1991). This sometimes results in the journal that has been 'produced' over the weekend before it has to be submitted rather than written over a period of time. One means of preventing this is to request that journals come in over one night on occasions, and then, while no reading or marking needs to be done, the fact that they are being written can be checked. Alternatively, if it may be appropriate to consider that if a learner manages to produce an adequate journal in one weekend, with the right kind of content, maybe that is 'good enough' – it depends on the selection of assessment criteria.

Some learners have difficulty in focusing their writing, particularly in the early stages of using a journal. 'Rambling' entries can be a problem, particularly where no structure is provided (Francis, 1995). Some learners recognize the role that rambling around ideas works for them. We have already cited Canning (1991) who reports one of her students as saying 'I just ramble until all of a sudden two or three words will fit together and key something. Then I realize that's it! That's where I'm having the problem! And then I can go with that.' Francis (1995) found those who rambled 'tended to assume stronger ownership of both the journal and the knowledge generated there'.

However, rambling can imply 'going in circles' or taking a superficial approach (Hoover, 1994; Ghaye and Lillyman, 1997). It may mean that learners are 'stuck' at the stage of descriptive writing and not actually progressing towards reflective thinking processes to reach useful outcomes of learning or more material for reflection. They may need help to understand how to 'move on' through the process.

Journal-writing activities may have a good chance of evolving positively but the project may also grow stale and the writing and the management of it may become a chore. This may be the time to put journals aside (Dillon, 1983; Wetherell and Mullins, 1996; Ghaye and Lillyman, 1997) or redesign the whole approach – or, as Shepherd (2004) says – 'the process of journal keeping must be enjoyable if it is to work well'.

Thinkpoint

Patrick Hutton quotes from the writings of Robert Stephen Hawker, a vicar in a remote coastal area of Cornwall, who did much to help the many shipwrecked sailors of that area and who taught his parishioners to bring the bodies back for Christian burial.

> I firmly believe that the daily affairs of us all are discussed among spirits and angels, and are helped or hindered by this as usually as one earthly friend helps another. The angels hear what we say, read what we write. One is looking over my shoulder now.
>
> (Hutton, 2004: 93)

Hawker wrote what were described as 'Thought books' which were helpful in supplying material for his sermons.

Chapter 10

Assessing journals and other reflective writing

Introduction

This chapter is primarily concerned with situations where journals are used in formal educational situations and where they are assessed, though initially we also deal with the question as to whether they should be assessed.

A little reflection on the subject matter of this chapter by the writer may be helpful to the reader. When the first edition of this book was being written (during 1998), the assessment of learning journals was an issue that still felt unsatisfactory, and while this chapter was an attempt to gather the current thinking of the time, there was a sense that there was more to be said on the matter – we had not 'cracked' the issue of assessment of journals. This second edition of the book covers progress in subsequent thinking. The chapter begins in a similar manner to the first edition, but the body of the chapter makes some different suggestions to those of the first edition. These new ideas have emerged mainly in the context of workshops and in the development of the work in Chapter 4 on the quality and depth of reflection (Moon, 2004a: Chapter 11 on Assessment). Structural issues around the concept of assessment are dealt with in Moon, 2002. The new ideas are initially introduced in the second section under 'Should journals be directly or indirectly assessed?'

'Assessment' is a word that is used differently in different situations. Here we take it to mean the review of a journal by others in order to determine whether it is adequate for the purposes set or to grade it. Adequacy or grade will be judged against a set of criteria that should have been set in advance, and which should be known by the writers of the journals. We have talked of the effect on the writing of a journal if the journal is to be seen by another – especially an assessor. Self-assessment avoids this second issue. A third topic of this chapter is the nature and quality of feedback that is given by the assessor to the learner.

Assessment of journals may be formative or summative. Formative assessment is a means of presenting learners with feedback on their work as they progress with it. It is more about learning than the usual notion of assessment. Summative assessment occurs at the end of the work and provides an overview of the quality of the work, sometimes as a grade or mark based on published criteria. We would understand assessment criteria for an assignment such as a journal to be related closely to the stated learning outcomes for the module or course.

Should journals be assessed?

There are many who argue that journals and reflective writing should not be assessed. A convinced proponent of journals in drama, Sister Therese Craig, asks:

> How can you mark an individual's own personal development? I think it's a right and proper part of education for us to encourage students to express their feelings so that they know it's all right to have those feelings. However, for me to mark those feelings seems inconsistent and incongruent. Marks can also create a barrier or obstacle to the person finding his or her own voice.
>
> (Dillon, 1983)

Sumsion and Fleet (1996) question the assessment of reflection in more general terms. They found that they faced the issue that underlies much of the content of this chapter – that of finding a suitable set of criteria by which to code the 'reflectiveness' of the students' work. They reviewed and rejected a number of instruments which were either too complex for the number of scripts with which they were working, or were composed of too many categories to obtain sufficient inter-coder reliability. They finally used criteria based on Boud *et al.* (1985). Despite the relative simplicity of their three-point scale – non-reflective, moderately reflective and highly reflective – their inter-coder reliability was only 50 per cent. As a result they say: 'at present, there are substantial difficulties involved in attempting to identify and assess reflection. Given current methodological and pragmatic limitations, the assessment of reflection raises complex issues of consistency and equity, as well as broader pedagogical and ethical concerns.' They abandoned their attempts to assess reflection.

It is very easy to go along with arguments that assessment of reflective writing or journals is intrusive on personal development or is too difficult because we cannot find the right critieria. However, there are reasons why we do need to develop means of assessment. The first reason reiterates the comments made by Sumsion and Fleet. Students are being assessed on journals and reflective writing even if marks are not being given. Even where journal-writing is assessed on the basis of 'competent' or 'not yet competent', or pass or fail/not yet pass, criteria being used – even if they are 'gut reactions' or personal interpretations and are never made explicit. When reflection and reflective practice are so highly esteemed in some areas of education and professional development, we should be able to do better than this. The coders involved in the work of Sumsion and Fleet demonstrated a substantial mismatch in their coding even when working with a simple scheme. One reason for this might be the lack of clarity of the assessment criteria (that they were simple does not mean that they were clearly defined). A second reason is that the purpose for the journal may not have been defined and discussed with the coders. A third is that the coders may not have been sufficiently 'educated' in the codes used. When a judgement is made about one item being better than another, criteria are used and we should be able to work with those criteria. There is not one thing called a journal and therefore unless there is clear guidance, different people will use different criteria.

The second justification for a system of assessment is based on the observation that even able learners may not find reflective writing in a journal easy (Wildman and Niles, 1987). Unless teachers have an understanding of the task that they are setting and the qualities in it that constitute a good performance, they will not be able to help these learners. As teachers, their ability to help may be hampered by the likelihood that they are (personally) naturally reflective and perhaps less able, thereby, to recognize the problems of others. The understanding of the task which teachers need in order to be helpful is displayed in their ability to work with criteria that distinguish quality from inadequacy – and these will coincide with assessment criteria.

A third justification for the assessment of reflective writing is rooted in the nature of the higher education system, as it seems to exist. The rise of the 'strategic' student is well documented (e.g. Kneale, 1997). 'Strategic students' are intent on success in their studies for the minimum output and will therefore not put effort into tasks that are not assessed. If we believe that journals contribute to learning, and we know that students will not maintain them unless they are assessed, then we need to assess them in some way. This will not be the case for all students – some will understand that there can be value in a task even if it is not assessed.

Fourth, we do now have typologies that can help with the production of assessment criteria for the quality of reflection – for example the generic framework for reflective writing (Resource 2).

The fifth reason for developing methods of assessing journals is the opposite of the tentative justifications above. Students are assessed on their programmes of learning and there is nothing wrong with setting journal-writing or similar work as a method of assessment (Paulson et al., 1991), and even as a method of grading students. What matters, as elsewhere, is that both teachers and the students are clear about the criteria for the assessment.

A sixth reason for the assessment of journals is that the process of assessment can enhance the learning that the learner does in the process of journal-writing. This point is linked to the new suggestions in this chapter that involve secondary reflection.

The last point is more general. Assessment does not always mean marking. In the sense that Brockbank and McGill use the term, it can mean 'sitting beside', a collaborative rather than an inspectorial system (Brockbank and McGill, 1998: 100–1). It is a helpful process to learners and it can bring structure and discipline to the work that might not come about in completely unassessed situations (Macrorie, 1970).

The points above strongly justify the development of assessment criteria for reflective and journal-writing even if they do not argue specifically for the necessity to mark or grade journals under all circumstances. The next section of this chapter follows on from this to consider issues and decisions that contribute to the design of assessment procedures.

Issues and decisions in the assessment of journals and reflective writing

Purpose

As usual, we suggest that the first guiding factor in terms of an assessment of a journal is the open declaration of the purpose for which the journal was set. Is the journal designed to enhance reflective practice, to enable the learning of something (content), to support creative thinking, or to help a learner's writing skills? The purpose should guide the decisions about assessment techniques and the criteria that are used.

What is to be assessed – process or product?

Whether the concern for the journal work is process or product or both is a matter that should be reflected in the statement of purpose for the journal, but it is an important question that is often not asked. Generally speaking, journal-writing employs reflective writing in order to support some form of learning. In many situations the learning is what is important, and the reflective writing is a means to that end. For example, Selfe *et al.* (1986) describe the use of journals with mathematics students. The aim of the work is not to develop reflective skills in these students, but to improve their learning. The quality of their reflection is incidental. At other times, the quality of the reflective process evidenced in the writing is at least as important as the learning that results. There are many examples in the literature of learning journals used in teacher education where the objective will be to enhance the skills of reflection on practice as well as to bring about learning. The work of Calderhead and James (1992) with the Record of Student Experience (ROSE) exemplifies this approach. While many, perhaps most uses of journal-writing will be expected to provide process and product outcomes, clarity about what is expected will guide the decisions about assessment. In situations where it is the learning that is important, there is much less of a problem with the development of criteria and the procedures. The learning may be evidenced directly in the journal and it is likely to be couched in disciplinary terms (Brockbank and McGill, 1998), or the learning may be assessed indirectly in examinations or other forms of assessment. The complexities of the assessment of journals become most evident when there is concern for the process as well as or more than the learning product.

Whether the journal is designed to enhance a process of reflective learning or the learning of some content (product), this should be reflected very clearly in the assessment criteria – and should be communicated to students very early on as part of the instructions about writing the journal.

Do we grade work or indicate the adequacy or inadequacy of it?

Learning journals might seem to be a departure from conventional forms of assessment, and we have already seen some of the difficulties in deciding the criteria. This latter difficulty does not go away if we decide to allocate simpler criteria and say that a journal is a pass or not yet a pass (or it is a fail) – but it is a great deal simpler. On the whole it is learners who want to be graded. Even if they know that they have 'passed' there is likely to be a wish to know how good the journal is in relationship to the criteria – or to other journals in the class. So there may need to be comments made about 'how good' and these should be based on some notion of what 'goodness' is in relationship to the purpose given in the first place. Grading requires greater definition of the criteria – and may raise some of the more difficult issues about agreement among different markers.

Who develops the assessment criteria?

The assumption is usually that it is teachers who develop assessment criteria. This does not have to be the case, and much learning can be achieved if learners themselves have a part to play in this process. A method of engaging learners might be to set the journal with an ascribed purpose and some very general guidelines that are based on general critiera. It should be allowed to 'run' for a while to let the learners become accustomed to working in the journal – and to deepen their reflection (Chapter 4). When the process is running smoothly, and the learners feel somewhat at ease with it, they are asked to use their own experience in order to work on the development of assessment criteria. Burnard (1988) suggests a method by which this may be done. Tutor and student 'brainstorm' criteria for assessment and from the list, each use the criteria in order to assess the journal and they make notes in support of their decisions. A discussion follows and a mark can be produced as a result of the discussion if necessary. In a method like this, criteria might best be developed at around a third of the way though the lifespan of a journal task, so the journals are only assessed during the second two thirds of the time.

Is the journal to be assessed by written work or other methods?

Most journals are assessed by written work – but there are several examples of oral assessments in the literature. In these cases, the examiners may have read the journal or may relate their questions to the material on which the journal is based. Martin (1998) has suggested that in this kind of interview, the more the learners are able to take control of the conversation, the more ability they are demonstrating in reflection.

Lindberg (1987) describes what he calls a 'conference' with his English literature students. The three conferences on the course are one-to-one, and they last around 15 or 20 minutes. Lindberg describes them to his students:

Since the journal is your gesture of making meaning, I will not grade it directly or read through it systematically. Instead, I want to respond to your own responses to what is going on in the journal. You'll summarize for me the high points of your journal and interpret yourself as an interpreter. And I'll probably ask you some hard questions about your responses and name for you what I see in your summary.

(Lindberg, 1987: 121)

He goes on to describe a longer (half-hour) conference at the end of the course in which performance is graded. The grade counts for a third of the marks of the course and the rest is made up of interpretive essays, which often relate to the material of the journal.

Should the journals be directly or indirectly assessed?

We explained at the beginning of the chapter that this chapter in this edition of the book is crucially different from that in the first edition. This difference is in the decision whether to assess the journals themselves or to assess a secondary piece of work that draws on the journals. Whether it is the journal or another piece of work that is assessed, there is still the need for the same considerations about assessment criteria. The secondary piece of work is likely to be a 'report' or 'account' (it is preferable not to use the term 'essay'). Depending on the purpose of the journal – the account may require the student to describe what she has learned as a result of working with the journal, often by citing examples or quoting from the journal. It may be required that the journal is submitted at the same time as the account, though this may counter the reasons for setting the secondary work. Asking students to hand in the journals means that there is an incentive to write an ongoing journal and properly to quote from it. Where learners have not been required to show evidence of working with a journal over a period of time, they have sometimes either written the 'journal' at the same time as the account – or not done it at all. It is possible to set up a system where a minimal mark is allocated to the journal that comes in alongside the account (e.g. up to 5 per cent) or to add a few marks (to the mark for the account) for excellent journals and take off a few for inadequate journals – though the quality of a journal should also be represented in the mark for the account.

The position taken in this chapter is now that the assessment of secondary material is usually the preferable choice. There are many reasons for this. The first is particularly important – we have said elsewhere that it is always advantageous to require a learner to go back over the material in reflective writing or a journal and go through a process of secondary reflection. In effect, the production of an account that is based on a journal requires this process of secondary reflection – and therefore the learner is likely to learn more from the process of using a journal when an account is marked. In effect it changes the role of a journal in a module or course from an assessment method to a tool for learning. Tools for learning can be freer and more exploratory and experimental if they are not the material that is actually assessed. Journals in this mode can almost be seen as equivalent to lecture notes.

There are other reasons for preferring the system of marking an account.

- We have cited a number of reasons why it may not be appropriate to mark very personal material in a journal. This system avoids the problem.
- Teachers often find the marking of conventional account more easily handled than the 'marking' of a journal even if the assessment criteria are clear.
- It can be easier for learners to draw in relevant material from elsewhere and relate it to their journal notes in an account than in an actual journal.
- Issues that can distract from fair assessment such as the format and presentation of a journal are removed from the situation.
- The issue of length of the material to be assessed can be more easily controlled.

We must reiterate that the purpose that the journal fulfils in the module or course must be considered in any consideration about the nature of assessment of the journals or accounts.

While we favour indirect assessment of learning journals, there are some remaining issues to discuss over the direct assessment of journals.

The management of the direct assessment of journals

Assessment of journals without direct grading

Assessment of journals does not automatically imply that the journal is allocated a grade. There are a number of alternatives to consider even in a modular system and bearing in mind the need to motivate the strategic student. First, the submission of a journal that meets some general characteristics of completeness and quality of presentation may be deemed essential for progression to the next modules, semester or year of study. Similar to this in its effect is the allocation of a single and fairly high mark to all journals that are adequate, with inadequate journals being returned for further work. A slightly more elaborate method is to use a system of three grades with simple assessment criteria such as length and regularity of entry distinguishing between them (e.g. Brodsky and Meagher, 1987). A different but equally simple approach is used by Jensen (1987) for physics students. The students were told that a well-kept journal, with quantity as the main criterion, could improve their semester course grade by up to a third of a grade point (e.g. from C to C+). This served to motivate 90 per cent of the students.

The assessment of journals within the context of a programme

Where marks are allocated to journals, there is a decision as to what percentage of the total programme or module mark will be given to the journal. There are a number of comments about this in the literature. Often those who have allocated a low percentage (for example around 10 per cent) have done so initially in order to ensure that journals are kept (Hahnemann, 1986). However, it appears to be relatively common for these percentages to be increased, sometimes quite dramatically, as the assessors have become more confident of the journal's contribution to learning and of their own ability to assess such work. For example, Brodsky and Meagher shifted percentages of course marks in a political science programme from 10 per cent to 75 per cent, having moved from initially seeing journals as an 'adjunct to, rather than an integral part of the courses' (1987: 375) and November shifted from a 10 per cent proportion to 40 per cent and a year later again he abandoned all other assessment, making the journal account for the total mark for his course. Hettich (1990) asked his students what percentage of total psychology course grades should be allocated to journal-writing. The median report was 25 per cent, which suggested that they preferred to see the journal as a 'supplement to other measures of learning'.

Coping with the volume of reading in the assessment of journals

An important issue in assessing journals directly is the potential issue of coping with the volume of reading that may arrive on the assessor's desk. If the assessment is formative as well as summative journals will be handed in for perusal and comment on a regular basis. It may be necessary to advise students either to restrain the volume of their writing, or to summarize material where original entries have been extensive. One mechanism that neatly overcomes the problem of reading volume is to ask learners to identify particular areas for summative assessment within the context of a complete journal. For example, they might be told that they should identify 2,500 words for assessment. This means that they have the opportunity to identify what they consider to be their best work, and the assessor reads less while being aware of the full journal (Houghton, 1998). There will need to be some form of annotation or page numbering system.

Developing assessment criteria for journals and for any reflective writing

In this section we do not present actual assessment criteria for reflection or for journals, but some examples that may be used for the development of assessment critera. In some cases, we present the references only. This is because there is no one view of purpose for a journal or for the nature of reflection. There are, however, many ideas around!

Some suggestions of general assessment criteria to indicate the adequacy of a journal

These criteria are derived from a range of sources in the literature, in particular Hettich (1976), Wagenaar (1984), Fulwiler (1987), November (1993). Most journals will need to demonstrate quality in at least some of the following:

- length
- presentation and legibility
- number of entries or regularity of entries
- clarity and good observation in presentation of events or issues
- evidence of speculation
- evidence of a willingness to revise ideas
- honesty and self-assessment
- thoroughness of reflection and self-awareness
- depth and detail of reflective accounts
- evidence of creative thinking
- evidence of critical thinking
- a deep approach to the subject matter of the journal
- representation of different cognitive skills (synthesis, analysis, evaluation, etc.)
- relationship of the entries in the journal to any relevant coursework, theories, etc.
- match of the content and outcomes of the journal work to course objectives, learning outcomes for the journal or purposes that the journal is intended to fulfil
- questions that arise from the reflective processes and on which to reflect further.

Assessment criteria developed from the frameworks of theory of others

While some of the schema below might seem attractive means to assess journal work, it is worth recalling the difficulties encountered by Sumsion and Fleet (1996) when they tried to use some more complex criteria for assessment of reflective accounts.

Criteria based on Bloom's taxonomy of educational objectives

Hettich (1976, 1990), using journals in the context of psychology courses, employs Bloom's (1956) taxonomy both as subject matter for the journal and as a means of analysis of the entries. This is described in Chapter 7. Hettich speculated that other models of thinking such as those of Perry (1970) and Belenky et al. (1986) might also contribute to the understanding of journal work.

Criteria based on King and Kitchener's model of reflective judgement

Ross (1989) developed a set of criteria for a teacher education programme. The criteria were not specifically developed to assess journal-writing, but various forms of reflective activities. Ross found that the seven-stage model of King and Kitchener (1981 – updated version, 1994) provides a good basis for development of criteria for assessing levels of reflection. The criteria are very much related to teacher education, but elements are extracted or summarized below in a more generalized manner.

Assessment based on the Structure of Learning Outcomes (SOLO) taxonomy

The SOLO taxonomy (Biggs and Collis, 1982) was developed as a means of describing the outcomes of learning and it has been used in a number of different contexts (e.g. Moon, 1999b). Davies (1998) used SOLO as a means of assessing student reports of art and design projects. The model consists of five levels that appear to be relatively easily recognized in written material. In Level 1 work (Prestructural), there is no appropriate structure to the task. The second level is Unistructural, with only one general element taken into account. In the third (Multistructural) level, there are several elements present in the representation but they are presented in an unrelated or poorly integrated manner. In the Relational (fourth) level, the several elements are integrated coherently in such a way that a new structure can be identified, but this new structure is not readily generalized to new situations. At the most sophisticated level – that of the Extended Abstract – the developed new structure is flexibly and competently generalized to new situations.

Assessment based on Van Manen's levels of reflectivity

Wedman and Martin (1986) used Van Manen's three schemata of levels to investigate the reflective abilities displayed in the journals of student teachers (Van Manen, 1977; Moon, 1999a). Van Manen's levels are:

• *Level 1*   Technical rationality: effective application of technical knowledge in order to reach known outcomes.

• *Level 2*   Practical rationality: teachers' ability to deal with practical actions where there are multiple factors in operation. There is an ability to cope with the confusion and make an assessment of the likely educational consequences.

• *Level 3*   In Wedman and Martin's terms, this level of critical rationality 'focused on incorporating consideration of moral and ethical criteria into discourse about practical action. The central question at this level was which educational goals, experiences and activities led toward forms of life that were just and equitable.'

It is interesting that there are again elements in common between this schema and the previous two. In Wedman and Martin's research, the contents of the 44 journals were analysed into thought units (Bales, 1957), and were then attributed to the three levels. All but four of the students demonstrated level 1 reflection; one was at level 2 and several appeared to be in transition between levels 1 and 2. The fact that they were in transition was taken to suggest that there is progressive development through the levels.

'Purpose-made' assessment tools: a 'framework for reflective thinking' as an assessment tool

This framework was developed for a pre-teaching programme that particularly promotes reflective approaches. It was developed in order to assess the effectiveness of the approach (Sparkes-Langer *et al.*, 1990; Sparkes-Langer and Colton, 1991). The framework is as follows:

- *Level 1*   no descriptive language
- *Level 2*   simple, layperson description
- *Level 3*   events labelled with appropriate terms
- *Level 4*   explanation with tradition or personal preference given as the rationale
- *Level 5*   explanation with principle or theory given as the rationale
- *Level 6*   explanation with principle/theory and consideration of context factors
- *Level 7*   explanation with consideration of ethical, moral, political issues

Again this framework, like those previously, provides a hierarchy of increasing complexity of material. In this case the research based on the framework did involve independent coders. Inter-coder reliability was 81 per cent (for matches no more than one level different) when the material was based on the ideas given in the framework. Reliability was less (not given) for the journal, 'possibly' because the format did not match the framework. The journal was subsequently modified to match the framework items. The need to alter the journal seems to be a considerable indictment of the framework. An assessment instrument for journal-writing or reflective writing would seem to require it to be of sufficient generality to cover the diversity of writing that can desirably result from a journal. There are some similarities between this approach and that taken later in this chapter.

Criteria for the recognition of evidence of reflectivity in writing

The work of Hatton and Smith (1995) arose from more thorough research than many of the studies described earlier. While the work derives from the context of teacher education, the descriptions of reflectiveness in writing are generally applicable. A summary of the framework with quotations from it is provided below:

• *Descriptive writing*   (which is considered not to show evidence of reflection) There is a description of events or literature reports. There is no discussion beyond description.

• *Descriptive reflection*   There is description of events but some justification in relatively descriptive language. The possibility of alternative viewpoints in discussion is accepted. Reflection may be 'based generally on one perspective factor as rationale' or, presumably in a more sophisticated form, is based 'on the recognition of multiple factors and perspectives'.

• *Dialogic reflection*   'This demonstrates a "stepping back" from the events and actions leading to a different level of mulling about discourse with self and exploring the discourse of events and actions'. Uses the 'qualities of judgements and possible alternatives for explaining and hypothesizing'. The reflection is analytical or integrative, linking factors and perspectives. It may reveal inconsistency 'in attempting to provide rationales and critique'.

• *Critical reflection*   'This demonstrates an awareness that actions and events are not only located within and explicable by multiple perspectives, but are located in and influenced by multiple historical and socio-political contexts.'

(Hatton and Smith, 1995)

The development of assessment criteria from the generic framework for reflective writing

To conclude this review of assessment criteria for reflective writing or journals, we go back to the model developed (Resources 2) as a means of helping students to learn to reflect. Since it represents a schema for quality and depth of reflection, it can serve as well as a source of assessment criteria in a similar manner to the work of Hatton and Smith. The levels might be taken as general criteria for quality or more finely divided criteria can be developed from the frameworks.

Giving feedback on the quality of journals

One issue about providing feedback to journal writers is to ensure that the teacher does not end up 'losing whole weekends buried in stacks of intimate scribblings' (Fenwick, 2001: 37). Fenwick sought ways of responding to the writers 'frequently and parsimoniously' and with sensitivity, acknowledging the 'frustrating craters of stuckness' and 'swampy bogs' into which journal-writing could thrust learners at times. The provision of feedback or the making of comments on journals requires greater sensitivity than other situations of marking. Sister Craig's comment about her students' feelings in the second section of this chapter epitomizes the issue. Cowan (1998b) suggests some very helpful guidelines for making sensitive comments on student journal entries:

- avoid writing comments in the first person in order to avoid setting up dialogue between writers and tutor when the dialogue should be between writers and themselves;
- avoid suggestion of judgements – provide an opportunity for writers to judge for themselves if it seems appropriate;
- ask a question or make a comment about a non-sequitur when it is useful to seek clarification;
- make a note when one wants to react negatively or positively to journal material but make no comment; however,
- indicate where more thinking could be appropriate or helpful.

Cowan stresses the responsibility of the assessor in overlooking journal material. The material should be treated as confidential and not discussed elsewhere.

Fenwick (2001) provides much helpful advice for those who respond to journals. She talks about the nature of response. It can be from a peer (e.g. in professional development situations), a supervisor or facilitator or the learner herself in a form of secondary reflection or review). Within those responses, there are different roles (Fenwick, 2001: 41):

- the comforter to the writer, boosting her strengths and widening issues towards more helpful perspectives;
- the mirror – reflecting and expanding the writer's own ideas;
- the provocateur – challenging and (carefully) being constructively critical;
- the learning director – helping the learner to make good use of what she is learning, and helping her to use useful directions;
- as friend-in-dialogue – sharing ideas in a conversational and gently supportive manner;
- as an evaluator – working to sharpen the learner's view, deepen her critical faculties. Fenwick indicates that the evaluator will be evaluating against agreed criteria;
- as a biographer – helping the learner to draw together the 'story' that the writer has told in the journal.

In addition to the possibly sensitive quality of the material in a journal, the purposes for which most journals are written would suggest a sense of ownership within which teacher comments may be physical impositions. Writing comments in pencil can partially overcome this. It is more gentle than the pen (in particular the red pen). Another method is to use yellow sticky notes or a page of comments referenced into the journal. Fenwick suggests that the use of a personal letter to the journal writer can be appropriate. Essential for this latter process to work would be clearly numbered pages or sections. Commenting on an audio-cassette tape which is given back to the learner is another useful possibility. It is a technique that is under-exploited for commenting on any assessed work.

Fenwick and Cowan make it clear that the response to something personal like a journal is not just feedback in the manner of most other assessments. More than other forms of assessment, it brings a range of dimensions of learning into active play: psychology, education, ethics and the politics of learning (Betts, 2004). It is important that issues such as these are considered by teachers who are going to be commenting on journals.

Some problem areas with journals and their assessment

A problem that we have already mentioned – that is almost inevitable, is that learners will tend to produce in journals what they think any assessor wants to see. They are, thank goodness, usually not stupid. Does this matter? It may not. In order to write what the tutor wants, they will have needed to go through a thought process that says 'I cannot write this – it would not be acceptable – or it would not get me good marks. I will modify it and make up a bit and make it seem like what I think is required.' That learner may, on the page, have concocted a version for the tutor – but in order to get there, she has gone through the appropriate reflection process, even if that does not get onto the page.

One problem that arises quite frequently with journals is that they are not written in an ongoing manner, but are written up at the last minute. This can be managed by occasional requirements that the journals are handed in overnight – not for marking. If the journal is not handed in, there may be marks deducted later – for example. An assessment criterion for a journal may be that there is adequate evidence of ongoing reflection. If a student can fake the 'ongoing-ness', maybe she is learning as much from the journal as if it were written as expected!

Plagiarism can be a problem – even though journal work or personal writing may be recommended as a means of counteracting it. Old journals can get around – and blogs are public material. Rothwell and Ghelipter (2003) had plagiarism problems and decided to slightly change the requirements of the journal task so that work from previous years could not be plagiarized.

Thinkpoint

Janette Rainwater is a therapist: in her book, she says:

> During my first hour with a new person I frequently will ask this seemingly nonapropos question: 'Which colour do you prefer, red, blue or black?' And

then I'll hand the startled person a book of blank pages bound in the colour of his choice. First of all it's fun to give a present to someone who's probably sitting there worrying about fees. Secondly it's thoroughly anti-psychoanalytic (giving a patient a gift? Come on!). Most important it is a concrete demonstration to the person of the value that I place on keeping a journal.

(Rainwater, 1983: 92)

Chapter 11

The enrichment and broadening of journal processes through the link with story

Introduction: definitions of story

This chapter is added to this new edition for two reasons – first because much work is being done in the area of story (or 'narrative') in education, professional activity and professional development that relates to and sometimes overlaps with that of the journal-writing process. Since we may choose to treat the journal as a collection of stories told usually from the first person, we can link the process of journal-writing in to the wider and sometimes different literature of the uses of story. Rich examples of the literature of story in particular disciplines are Greenhalgh (1998) – medicine, McDrury and Alterio (2003) – professional education in health, Kenyon *et al.* (2001) – gerontology.

The second reason for adding this chapter to a book on journal-writing is that the integration of story activity with journal-writing extends the value of the latter by widening its context from the world of the individual perception into the social, political and historical context of the individual. More generally, this chapter explores the relationships between the journal and story processes in order that they may helpfully enrich each other – for the influence goes both ways. We talk of plural relationships because there are different conceptions of what 'story' is, and many different journal activities.

We start by seeking some frameworks or definitions of story. A broad view of the definition of story allows it to extend from pure fiction and fantasy to the description of experienced events of a personal nature. The latter may coincide with what goes on in journal-writing, though there is some sense also that a story is a discrete event with a distinct beginning, a middle and a form of closure. 'Fact' and 'fiction' are not, of course, discrete categories. There is a logical argument that all fiction is generated on the basis of the inner experience of the writer and that we read it by matching it to our own inner experiences. The attribution of meaning even to a word has come about through experience. The processes of representation of an idea, of retelling it and of reading or hearing a story are all processes of interpretation – or reshaping (Lamarque, 1990) – which is, in its way, the development of new fiction. We again explore the ways in which fiction and experience are close in the discussion that follows the presentation of the framework (page 124).

The discussion above indicates that there may be no clear logic that divides story from journal-writing, and fiction from non-fiction so, in order to pursue this chapter further, we create an organizing framework for this discussion. We start by reminding ourselves that story can be written down or told, or depicted in cartoons, comic strips (Beard and Wilson, 2002) (or in cave drawings), though mostly we refer to the written word here. We are also going to make the assumption that the word 'story' is used when the material is to be shared with others or communicated. In this way it is usually different from journal-writing as the latter tends to be initially for the use of the writer even if it is shared with others. Another connotation of story is that it has some coherence and unity – a 'grasping together' (Ricoeur, 1984) – if not a beginning, middle and closure. In addition, in a journal a story may be spread across many entries, and it may never be written in a coherent 'one episode' story form. Another word for this might be 'theme'. Moreover, there are very likely to be stories within stories like Russian dolls . . .

Making sense of story in journal-writing: the development of a framework

In the framework, story is seen to consist of:

• *Personal story*   The description and/or reflection on specific incidents or events (critical incidents) that have some unity and coherence and link to the person's experience.

• *'Known' story told in a professional, workplace, educational or similar setting*   These are the stories told informally or formally among people who share experiences such as within a profession, workplace, or the within their role of learners on an educational programme and so on. The stories are about events or experiences that relate to the common interests of the tellers or those who listen.

• *Non-fiction but 'not personally known' story*   These are the material of education (elements of the curriculum) and the media. They are stories that are at a distance from the individuals, but they are taken to be 'true' or authentic accounts within a familiar experience or context (for example, of a shared profession or workplace). These are the stuff of case studies.

• *Fiction and fantasy*   Fictitious stories are those that are accounts of events which have not actually been experienced as happening as described. As we have said, fiction is made up of elements of experience and it is interpreted by the listener in relation to some elements of her experience.

• *Storytelling*   By this we imply the act of telling a story. We add this category because sometimes the very act of telling is more significant than the content. Storytelling is also a generic term that may be used to describe any kind of work with story.

With the vocabulary of story described in the framework, we make points that are relevant to the rest of the chapter, and then we can explore the more precise ways in which journals relate to the framework. The first point returns to the notions of fiction and non-fiction. This is important in relation to the argument (later) that there is a valuable but underexploited place for fiction in educational settings. The sense is made in the following way: one person's personal story become another's 'known story' when the first transmits it to another. When a person first communicates her story to a group, it is her experience and it becomes a known story to the group members. If members of the groups communicate the original 'known story' to another group, the story becomes the new group's non-fiction story – not known or personal – but an authentic story. An example of such a situation in professional studies might be where known stories of one group of professionals are communicated to another group as a series of case studies. To this latter group, whether the case studies were 'made up' (i.e. fiction) or were originally based on real-life situations probably does not matter. In addition, different people's view of the same story can seem like many different fictions (Whelan *et al.*, 2001).

The second general point that the framework enables us to make returns to the idea expressed earlier, that the use of story alongside journals 'widens the context from the world as perceived by the individual – into the social, political and historical context of that individual, or into a consideration of "otherness"', as Greenhalgh and Collard (2003) put it. Bruner (1990) talks of stories developing the 'outer landscape' which relates to action and the inner landscape that relates to thinking pocesses. The telling and hearing of myth, traditional and modern tales (even 'soaps' – Crossley, 2002) is a means by which we learn what it is to live in our present society (Claxton, 1999). Reflection in a journal tends to be seen as individually focused but linking journal-writing and story allows the experience of the individual to be related to that of others. It can be related to the idea of being within an organizaton or system or a social setting and to other aspects of the wider context of the individual's life – through the story of other situations and through fiction. The individual can go beyond her immediate experience, while using the common element of story to make the link. We use a quotation to illustrate and elaborate this point. It is not without significance that the quotation uses metaphor – a story – to explain itself:

> Stories are gatekeepers between our inner and outer worlds. The known world is the starting point, the connection with a reality which we can identify and recognise. In the process of its unfolding, the tale develops a story line which contains and explores the unknown. A story is a guide because it takes us from resting place to adventure, through misfortune to culmination and the end. The listener walks metaphorically, hand in hand with the storyteller, inside whom the tale finds a temporary abode. When the story is completed, we, the listeners, emerge revitalised. The imagination has nourished and inspired our motivation which, in turn, contributes to realisation and solution. We gain

strength by identification with the story character who had the will to persist and who found the courage and strength to prevail.

(Gersie and King, 1990: 35)

Journals in relation to the 'making sense of story' framework

We use the framework (above) to organize this middle section of the chapter.

Personal story

While we have said that this kind of story is, for the most part, the 'stuff' of journals, we do not tend to recognize or treat it in that way in a journal. Taking the view of a journal as a series of stories makes it possible to work with the material of a journal in new ways – for example, through the story/storytelling methods of a number of people who would not have seen themselves as working with journals as such (e.g. Bolton, 1994; Winter *et al.*, 1999; Bolton, 1999; McDrury and Alterio, 2003; Alterio and McDrury, 2003; Alterio, 2004; Drake and Elliot, 2005). Taking an incident in a journal as a story means that we can examine it in ways that are less encumbered by its context in the journal. Many of the techniques in Chapter 13 can be applied more easily. It is as if the incident, extracted as a story from a journal, can be turned over in the hands, examined from different sides, looked at from underneath or looked at afresh. It can be passed over to others for examination. We link here into other disciplines and consider what they can do with a personal story. The journal-based story can be enacted in drama where the provider of the story can learn from seeing it acted out, as can others (Neelands, 1992; Boal, 1995). Alternatively it can become the subject matter for development in creative writing (e.g. Hunt and Sampson, 1998; Hunt, 2000). It can be shared in the context of professional development (see below) or in the use of techniques that will enhance the reflective aspects of it (for example the use of 'critical friend' techniques).

'Known' story told in a professional, workplace, educational or similar setting

'Story' in a professional context usually involves the giving of accounts of actual personally related events that have been experienced in practice (Connelly and Clandinin, 1990; McDury and Alterio 2003), or stories told about practices in an organization (Snowden, 2003) or in an area of human interest and endeavour such as health and medicine (Greenhalgh and Collard, 2003). Some might not use the word 'story' for these situations but, perhaps, refer to them as 'critical incidents'. In terms of vocabulary, we would use the more technical term 'narrative' instead of 'story'.

To be relevant to this book on learning journals, we assume that the stories that form the known or unknown are either the product of journal-writing or other reflective learning, or the process of story is a means of enhancing the subsequent reflection on material that might be the subject matter of journals or other reflective methods.

The story method that is used by Alterio and McDrury (2003) fits this section, and we now describe it. An 'experienced story' is offered to a professional group – the story is told by the teller from her perspective. The listeners notice content and emotions, but do not interrupt. There is then a stage of clarification of the story, questions are asked and points may be expanded with links made to prior experiences of listeners or the teller. This moves into a stage in which the material of the story is drawn out to show how the perspectives of others may relate to the content. There is then critical questioning in order to analyse the role of assumptions or prior experiences which have led the teller and listeners towards their various interpretations of the story. 'Key players' in the story are identified and randomly allocated to the whole group which then acts out the story. The aim of this is to 'provide the teller with a range of alternative ways to examine (her) story' (p. 49). There is a debriefing and room for further reflection. Bolton (1999) provides an example of similar work with a known story, and suggests the following as some of the other exercises which can be undertaken that enable those working with a narrative to 'get into the story':

- writing what a character might be thinking at a particular point;
- writing what might be a diary entry for a character;
- interviewing a character on paper;
- transcribing an imagined phone conversation from one character to another at a particular point in the story.

Other story techniques in organizations differ. Snowden (2003) describes the use of story in organizational situations. Sometimes an expert in story work may collect and retell stories to an audience, or she may use established myth as a means of eliciting story. He points out that the stories about the organization that tend to be put around by the management are of the 'Janet and John' type (or cultural equivalents). He says 'The trouble with Janet and John is that they are just too good; they make any self-respecting and intelligent child sick.' The real stories need to be drawn from those who make up the workforce. Also in the organizational context, that of Hewlett Packard, Nymark (2000) sought to understand the stories that 'constitute the understanding of the company's culture' (p. 2), how these stories related to everyday practices and how they could be used for the company's general benefit. He suggests that stories in organizations can form a social map that may be used by new employees, for example in the manner that the stories 'point out both the dangerous and the safe areas' (p. 56). They help employees to make decisions on their own, and to increase their understanding – thus reducing supervision needs.

In the context of higher education, another example of this process is described by Linden (1999), who collected stories from supervisors of PhD students. In the course of the first of a two-day seminar on supervision issues 444 stories were collected. Some were written from the viewpoint of the supervisor, some from the viewpoint of the students. The scripts of the stories were then used as the basis for the learning in the second day, in which the aim was to sensitize the supervisors to issues that affected their students.

Non-fiction but 'not personally known' story

We have pointed out that once a 'personally known' story is passed on to another and repeated, it is 'not personally known'. It may be presented as case study material or as an anecdote or as research findings that may be used to educate others.

The first example returns to the work of Linden (1999) whose work is described above. The workshops on the experiences of supervisors were one outcome of the work, but also formed the basis for work on competence development for the further training of supervisors. This removed the stories from their personal context, and used them in a different manner.

Greenhalgh and Collard (2003) describe the use of story in the health service and demonstrate their methods in a workbook that centres on the learning about diabetes care by multi-professional groups. The material used was developed by a group of health workers with responsibility for the management and health outcomes of diabetes in a Bangladeshi community. They typified situations and issues that were encountered. The stories were used by other groups to whom the material was, in effect, non-fictional case story. They focused on themes such as diagnosis, loneliness and lack of support. Methods for the work with the stories are suggested and the aim was a change in the practice of participants.

In other situations the material generated by the telling of stories may be used to inform the literature of the subject matter, and that in turn can be used to inform the writing of those who are using learning journals. Sparkes (2002) illustrates this approach in a thorough manner. He looks at and illustrates with examples, the many sources of tales in sport and the manner in which they contribute to qualitative research. He looks at many approaches including the scientific tales, realist and confessional tales, poetry, drama and fictional sources.

Fiction and fantasy

We have said that once the source of information is unknown by the recipient of the information, whether it is 'fact' or 'fiction' may not matter if the aim is to learn from the material. The fictionalizing of case material may be a deliberate process to meet ethical requirements – but here the focus is not on fictionalizing as a means of necessary disguise, but it is on the deliberate and positive use of 'made-up' material. There will be tensions between those who would declare that the 'made up' is 'only imagination' and therefore has no place in formal education or professional development – and those, like the present writer, who would argue otherwise. Discussions about fiction, artistry and non-fiction are explored more fully in Hunt (2000: the conclusion) and in chapter 7 of Winter *et al.* (1999) which is subtitled 'The strange absence of the creative imagination in professional education'.

Fiction is 'free' – it can go anywhere, it can be used to make any point. It can be used to focus attention on specific issues or to pinpoint important but subtle issues for learning. It can also work freely with emotional material that may not be possible with 'real-life' stories, they can enhance affective learning (Noddings, 1996). It can take us into the theorizing, the 'what if's', the 'supposing . . .' realms. Made-up stories can be twisted and turned to serve their purposes. New endings can be developed, removed and altered. This is achieved by way of using imagination. As Gersie and King (1990) say:

> The multi-dimensional quality of imagination makes it possible for us to reach the darkest corner of our being, to reveal our most hidden belongings and capacities . . . The multi-functional aspect of imagination helps to resolve, reconcile, energise, stimulate and encourage. In itself, the imagination is neither good nor bad, it is the function which we give to it which determines its usefulness.
>
> (Gersie and King, 1990: 36)

There is much untapped potential in the use of fiction in the role of providing support and enrichment for work in learning journals. We survey some of these roles and relevant literature under separate headings even though there are overlaps between them.

We can learn more about a topic by working with it in fiction

The writer was interested in the issue of confidentiality of journal-writing in a relationship. Writing a fictitious story about a journal-writer in a relationship expanded her thinking on the matter. Overtly the story was fiction – but there were many elements of autobiography that were bound up in it. The fiction allowed the issue of confidentiality of personal writing to be picked up, turned over in the hands and explored relatively free from the constraining ties of 'what really happened' in particular instances (Moon, 2005b).

Mansfield and Bidwell (2005) talk of the use of fiction as a means of 'illumination and increasing the understanding' of research processes. They work with a group of Master's level students on a Community Education programme – and say that their students come onto the programme with a belief that they will be told to 'write themselves out' of their inquiries. Instead, the use of story, creative writing techniques and 'reflexive journals' enable them to 'regain trust in their own senses', to 'unlock their creativity and enable them to re-enage as autonomous learners with a range of ways of knowing and furthermore to recognise that research is not only an epistemological activity but also an ontological one'.

Winter *et al.* (1999), working in the field of professional development, discuss the use of short stories as a means of capturing the 'uncertainty, instability, uniqueness and value conflict' (p. 3) which Schön (1983, 1987) has done so much to characterize as central issues in professional work. Winter *et al.* also describe the development of 'patchwork texts' as a means of exploring topics in professional development. They characterize a patchwork text as broader than story. While a story aims to conclude or round off (that is, have an ending), a patchwork text is ongoing and open-ended. It is made up of a range of pieces of writing, some of which may be fiction. The aim is that the pieces have relationships to each other, in providing contrasting perspectives on a topic, in different modes. There is room for art, philosophy, science, academic writing – anything – with the unities existing in the individual pieces as well as overall. In practice in the academic programme, the writers indicate that the patchwork texts tend to consist of five or six pieces of writing of around a page long and there may be a fairly brief reflective commentary. It is interesting to note that assessment criteria for the work match closely the characteristics for the taking of a deep approach to reflection (see Resources, 2: A generic framework for reflective writing).

The exploring of 'what ifs?', 'supposing . . .'

Progoff (1975) was interested in the energy left in paths not taken – decisions that have led to no change – but from which we can move into looking at possible future scenarios. One way of entering into this kind of story-writing is to take an event described in a journal and to alter one element of it. In Chapter 7, the writer has explored the use of imagination to enhance the learning from short courses and workshops – so that on the course, learners anticipate how things will be when they put the new ideas from the course into practice. To explore these anticipations is to write fiction – and whether the fiction is written with known characters or not does not matter – there will be different learning from either approach.

The use of story to explore and stimulate thinking on a topic

The use of story here may be the reading of fiction. Gough (1993) argues that the reading of science fiction and postmodern texts model human interrelationships with the environment and understandings of 'nature' and 'reality' more effectively than much of the expository scientific writing. A similar idea is put forward by Gundmundsdottir (1995) who talks of the use of stories from different cultural perspectives. In both of these case, a logical intermediate form for the musings brought about in learners as a result of such reading of fiction is the learning journal – that can serve as a place for the sense-making process.

The use of guided imagery to broaden thinking

The use of guided imagery is another manner in which there can be a relationship between journal-writing and fiction (Beard and Wilson, 2002). Guided imagery techniques usually use an initial 'lead-in' which induces relaxation and then they 'take' the listener to an imaginary situation from which the listener is invited to progress with the story-line in some manner which is generated by their imagination rather than being driven by decision-making processes. Such work may be preceded and followed by journal activities – and/or linked with the topic of the journal-writing.

Storytelling

Storytelling is different from the other categories because it can encompass any or all of them. In this account we seek it as the act of making the story public and available to the senses of others. This is the activity described in several story initiatives that are mentioned earlier in this chapter. We have talked of the difference between reflection and the representation of reflection. When a story is first written there is a process of representation of the thinking/reflective processes that constitute the cognitive activities. We have said that there is learning from the process of representation. When a story is then told there is a further opportunity for the teller to learn from the story. She may need to reformulate it if it is to be told orally (i.e. not from direct reading), but even if the story is read, it then becomes available to others to provide reactions, give feedback, twist and turn and develop the ideas in order that a whole group may learn more from the story. In this way storytelling can extend the value of story writing for the writer – and hence the value to the journal writer.

We have made the case in many different ways that the use of fiction and non-fiction – the writing or reading of stories – has much to contribute to work in journals. The skilled use of story lies in the manner of its introduction and the creative and sensible presentation of purpose in such a way that it deals with the learner's question, 'How is this going to help us to learn?' Beyond this it is pertinent to say that story is attractive and by nature engaging to learners.

Thinkpoint

This extract is from a commercial storytelling organization in the USA, which sends 'e-tips' on storytelling by email to those who subscribe (for free). The text below is a little re-arranged but the meaning has not changed.

> Keep a story journal . . .
>
> . . . when an image or scene or story comes to you, honour it. Treat an unbidden image like an interesting stranger who knocks at your door. Show it respect. It may be offering you an invitation to a new adventure . . . Give imagery-thinking its place in the sun. When you are stalled in any endeavour, take a moment to consult your imagery mind. Ask yourself for an image that will help you. Notice whatever image comes and pay attention to it . . .

Alternate between linear thinking and imagery thinking. Follow your logical thoughts as far as they lead you and then try to notice if there is an image waiting in the wings . . .

Develop your abilities to communicate images.

(Lipman, 2003)

Chapter 12

Examples of journals

Introduction

This part of the book aims to provide some ideas that will enhance any journal-writing in general. This chapter, in particular, moves away from the viewing of parts of journals to take a look at several examples of whole journals or methods of using journals. The next chapter will provide a range of activities that can be used in any journal or other forms of reflective writing.

The journals or journal methods illustrated in this chapter are chosen because they are mentioned in earlier parts of the book, for reference and information and for interest. The aim of the chapter is to provide ideas, guidance and the encouragement to get involved in an area of writing in which the possibilities are boundless. We have not included in this chapter journals that are specifically designed to support discipline learning in higher education courses because the better descriptions of these tend to have been included earlier.

The first two examples represent methods of using journals as well as discussion of journal format. The first is the Intensive Journal of Progoff, to which reference has been made in many parts of this book. The second is a description of a manner of using journals as a support to the learning in training and short courses. The third example describes a form of a journal that has a strong function as an organizer of personal activity as well as a means of support and development of personal learning. The next is the format of journal that the writer has evolved as a personal development journal over many years of use. Alongside the personal journal, there is an example of a project journal. The project, in this case, is this book. The last case study is again of a journal to which a number of references have been made in the text. It is a journal that was developed by Morrison (1990, 1996) to accompany learning on a modular postgraduate programme.

Progoff's Intensive Journal

Progoff's background is of significance in understanding his development of the Intensive Journal because his orientation influenced the structure of the journal

(Progoff, 1975). Progoff, for example, studied under Carl Jung for a time. He was also one of the founders of the Association for Humanistic Psychology but was neither a therapist nor only a psychologist as such. Kaiser (1981) describes him as a philosopher theologian alongside Buber and Tillich. Similarly to them, Progoff was interested in the meaning that people could make of their lives and the events that confront them. The spiritual element is clear in the nature of the text of the books that Progoff wrote about the journal and its processes and in the nature of the workshops that are designed to introduce the journal (Progoff, 1975, 1980). The workshops are described alongside the journal structure in Progoff (1975).

The Intensive Journal itself consists of 19 sections in which the journal writer works. Progoff describes this form of the journal as representing: 'An instrument . . . capable of drawing together the multiplicity of contents of human life, [and] compressing them into a more manageable space while not losing the quality of movement and change that is their essence' (1975: 21). The structure evolved both from his research work in depth psychology where he was concerned with people's life histories, and from his therapeutic work.

Each section in the Intensive Journal is associated with a particular type of subject matter and/or with particular methods of writing. A number of the methods of working are described in the last chapter (Chapter 13) as activities. Examples of the sections are 'daily log' (recording of daily events), 'dream log' (for record-ing dreams) and 'dialogue' sections (a number of sections that are related by the use of a dialoguing method). On any occasion writers might start by recording in the daily log section and move from there to work on other aspects of their current experience in different ways in other sections, always cross-referencing the entries. Another time they might start with a section that is associated with a form of activity that generates memories to explore further ('Footprints' see Chapter 13). There is also a 'life-history log' for material that relates to the writer's previous life story. These descriptions may be specific or they may represent brief memories that have arisen in connection with writing in another part of the journal. Another interesting section is 'intersections' (see Chapter 13). This relates to 'roads taken and not taken' (1975: 145) – to decision points in life where a decision is made to take one course of action as opposed to another. Progoff suggests that there can be value in examining the decision not taken as there may be matters still of value to learn.

There is a concept of 'flow' that underlies the Intensive Journal. By flowing between the past, present and future and across different sections of the journal, the writer integrates the various elements of his or her life and develops a greater sense of self – 'who I am'. We have mentioned that Progoft's journal has been used effectively with unemployed groups and it has had frequent use in situations of spiritual development or exploration. In both these groups the development of personal identity is important.

Unfortunately, the book, written by Progoff, that describes the use of the Intensive Journal is not very accessible, being written in a ponderous and meditative mode to accompany and match the atmosphere of the workshops (1975). Other literature that interprets Progoff's work is actually a better introduction to the methods, although it loses something of the spiritual nature of the whole experience of attending a workshop and continuing to write in the recommended style. Examples of useful and reasonably comprehensive references to Progoff's work are Rainer (1978), Miller (1979), Kaiser (1981), Cell (1984), Hallberg (1987), Burnham (1987) and Lukinsky (1990), among others.

Using journals to support learning in short courses

The origin of this work was the writer's involvement in professional development in the health service (health promotion). The work role involved the development of short training courses, largely for nurses, of one or two days or slightly longer. There was a concern that it was all too easy for participants to sign on and to attend the course – and then to go back to their workplace and do nothing different. The course did not have impact. There might be several reasons for this. The course might have been taught badly, the participant might not have found it relevant, but often it seemed that the reason was that the new behaviour suggested in the course was not sufficiently linked into the participants' current behaviour patterns. Back in the workplace, with work piled up from the day or two on the course, it was easier for participants to put the ideas on one side ('for when I have more time to think about it all') and to carry on with old patterns. It became evident that this was a pattern that was true for many courses in many other contexts.

One approach to increasing the impact of short courses is to specify the improvement of practice in terms of anticipated learning outcomes, instead of being concerned only with the learning that should be achieved in the training period (Moon, 2002). Developing from this is the need to embed the ideas by developing plenty of time for reflection in the period of the course. However, just reflecting on the content of the course is not sufficient. There needs to be consideration of how the new ideas fit into the current practice and can result in changed or improved practice. It is a process that needs imagination and reflection – and still this is not all. The knowledge that professionals such as nurses and teachers have of their practice tends to be tacit and often not readily expressed or modified without some encouragement (Schön, 1983).

On a short course there is little time or opportunity for participants to learn new ideas and go through these various stages of embedding the ideas into their understanding of their practice. This is where journals are useful – even for one-day courses. The writer developed the following framework as a structure that can underpin the reflective writing that goes into a journal and it serves to guide the sequence of a course as well (Moon, 2004c). It is divided into four phases:

• *Phase 1*   An awareness of current practice with regard to the subject matter of the course is developed.

• *Phase 2*   The content of the new learning is clarified and related to the current understandings.

• *Phase 3*   The new learning is considered in relationship to the current practice.

• *Phase 4*   There is anticipation and imagination of the nature of the changed/ improved practice. It will be based on the question 'What will you do that is different tomorrow?'

Journal-writing that roughly follows this sequence or that uses it as an underpinning structure is likely to facilitate the embedding of the new ideas into practice. During the course, there will be periods for reflective activity. These periods may involve pairing off and talking about the material that has just been presented and then making journal entries on the basis of discussion, or they may involve just writing.

It is hard to achieve much change of practice in a course that lasts for one day. However, the reflective activity on a course can be extended. One method is by asking participants to do 'prework' before a course. A method of working with prework is to provide a set of up to five questions (around 15 minutes' work) which are designed to develop an appropriate mind-set to the material of the course before the participants arrive. It can incorporate questions about the current work practices. The prework represents the first entries into the journal and the facilitator might ask for one set of it to be sent so that she can integrate it into the course activities.

The extension of a course at the other end can be achieved by the requirement that participants produce some assignment task or a report in order to be 'signed off' or awarded a course certificate or university credit. The assignment may, for example, be a learning journal recording the process of instituting the change in practice or it might be a piece of writing that requires reference to an ongoing reflective account that relates to the impact of the course.

A 'daybook' that supports professional activity and learning

Over the past 14 years, the writer has used a daybook system to support her activity and learning in three different work situations. Most of the work was developmental, somewhat unpredictable and, in different ways, involved a multiplicity of networking and meetings with people in different locations or work. The daybook that is described here probably only just qualifies as a form of journal as it is on the edge of being record-keeping system – but there is some learning output and there is a section for reflective thinking. In terms of format, the writer used an A5 (or roughly half-letter size) loose-leaf file for the daybook, and that required cutting and punching A5 paper and making the section dividers. Personalizing even this professional activity book seemed to be important and it is covered in blue leather that helps also with wear and tear. The daybook contains the following sections (though obviously there is room for customizing here):

• In front of the first section there is spare paper (see later).

• *Records*   At times there has been a need to make lists of people for contact, the timetables for small projects and so on. In this section, the achievements of the contacts or the elements of the timetable can be recorded.

• *To do*   This is a vital section in terms of organization. The list develops and extends, with items crossed out as they are dealt with. Every so often the list is rewritten. Rewriting provides a sense of greater organization as the expansive list with many crossed-out items condenses back onto one, or two, pages. Sometimes the list splits into shorter- and longer-term matters.

• *Thoughts*   This is the reflective learning part of the daybook. It is the ongoing reflection, the capture of stray ideas that as yet have no home, the place for thinking through concepts, the playing with ideas which may then be lifted into a more permanent place outside the daybook or within. The section may be the home for the initial ideas for a project or the development of notes from a meeting. It is a section to wander through on occasions – on the bus or the train, keeping what is in there 'alive'.

• *Contacts and references*   This section is for making a quick note of work contacts, phone numbers and sometimes references. The material here may be lifted into a conventional diary or other place.

• *Meeting list*   This and the next section have been crucial to networking activities. The 'meeting list' section contains a list of all meetings that have been attended and phone calls where there is information that needs to be kept. The notes of the meetings/phone calls are filed in the next section (Meetings). The Meeting list provides a number for the meeting, the name of the person or group involved, and sometimes the location.

• *Meetings*   Here are filed the notes of meetings or significant phone calls. These will have been written on a homemade A5 clipboard. Each page is numbered (theoretically in red) with the same reference number that relates to the previous section. This section tends to fill up and then the notes are removed and stored separately. They are stored, bound with a treasury tag – but with dates and numbers still easy to locate from the Meeting list.

A format for a personal journal

In Chapter 1, I introduced my own journal-writing activity as a part of the introduction to this book. The personal journal does have that role and I would probably not be writing this book were it not for that personal enthusiasm. In this section I will be more objective about my own experiences in considering how they have led me to design and redesign formats for journals. Such a process does not seem unusual among journal writers. Rainer (1978) and Grumet (1990) are among others who describe 'evolutions'.

I go back now to the experience of learning to use Progoff's Intensive Journal, and the significance of that for my journal-writing habit. For a while I wrote in most of the 19 sections designated by the Intensive Journal, particularly while I was able to get to the series of associated workshops. Then, as with many of us who started on the Progoff system, the inability to sustain the effort overcame enthusiasm and the maintained sections tailed off towards a daily recording in the daily log, period and dream-log recording and occasional work in other sections. I also rapidly ran out of space in the A4/letter-sized file which was provided at the workshop and found that A5 pages were much more convenient and portable. I made two new sets of section dividers. One set went into a small personalized file for 'everyday' journal-writing and once a year or so, I would move the accumulation of journal material into a larger file. I found that the fat A5 files which had been produced to contain the weekly instalments of recipes or gardening hints povided a useful location for the long term stowage of journal material, and allowed the daily journal to be maintained at a reasonably portable size.

I maintained a journal regularly in this format, for many years and most of it still occurs but the format evolved once more. At this stage there was usually a bulging section for the daily log, entries in the period log and slim fillings for one or two other sections and little elsewhere. I continued to find particularly satisfying the period log – looking back over a period of time and considering it as a distinctive whole, with images and feelings that are associated with it but that are different from those of another period. It is intriguing to sense when a period of life is coming to an end and when, suddenly, there is a sense that a new period has begun. I also put into this section a copy of the letter I write each Christmas to friends. This is in the form of a period log whose timing is enforced by the pattern of the year. I write at the end of the day. It seems to take on the role of a closing down of the day, and in writing, I feel easy and settled.

In adopting this format, I confronted another issue. How would I deal with all the sections of the Intensive Journal, which I did still occasionally use? It was hard to change a habit of some 20 years, but I admitted to myself that I was not using the sections on a regular enough basis to maintain all the divisions and I needed to make the whole thing simpler. I arrived at a format of two sections only. One is the daily log. The other is a section for anything else – 'workings' I call it. It is a section for anything other than daily entry material – for dreams, for stray thoughts, journal activities, systematic 'thinking through' or for period log entries. These entries are dated and given a title and there is a cross-reference into the daily log section. In many ways, this system is relatively similar to that of Rainer with her 'diary tools' but both do rely on a working knowledge of a range of techniques that can be called into use when there is need or there is time to explore.

Most of the content of my journal has always concerned my emotional life, with relatively little concerning descriptions of events. This changed, however, when I was travelling. Then I would want to be descriptive and also I would not want to carry even the A5 file. I have several times, therefore, punched a number of sheets of paper and two pieces of stiff board, sandwiched the paper between the boards and used treasury tags to hold it all together. As a light travel journal, such arrangements have worked well and the paper has been re-filed with my normal journal on return. The travel log has now evolved to have an identity of its own and it is now a separate notebook, which has been halved again. It is an A6 sketchbook which contains sketches and text. I carry with it one coloured pencil that has a lead made up of five colours, and a pencil. The pencils and the book are in a small leather pouch – very convenient for travel.

Perhaps it was the stirring of thought about journals caused by the emerging notion of this book that gave rise to the next stage of evolution in which my habit is located at the present time. It is the format and not the content or sections of the journal that has changed. I decided that just writing at the end of the day, as a kind of summary activity, was not satisfactory any longer. I wanted to be able to write notes, descriptions of events, to think on the paper of my journal at any time. This posed problems of portability. My A5 file could not be carried easily because A5 would not fit into a convenient size of handbag. I did not want to reduce the paper size for this daily journal because I would have felt constrained by a very small page on which to write. I could have moved on to using a pocket organizer. I therefore decided to fold in half the A5 paper (to A6, or roughly quarter letter size) and protect it with two slightly larger than A6 boards that are jointed in the middle so that they fold over the folded paper (Figure 12.1). Treasury tags through holes in the paper and boards hold it all together. As with the daybook, personalizing a journal seems to be important. This journal's covers are suede and are held closed with a red band. There are only a few pages in the portable journal and

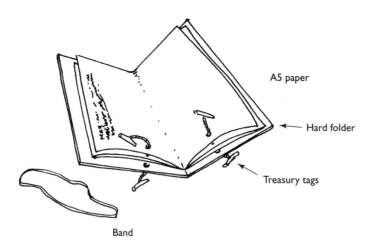

Figure 12.1 A portable A5, or roughly half-letter size, journal.

when a page is written on both sides, it is transferred into the old A5 file. This arrangement has proved to be relatively satisfactory. It is still in place as I write the second edition of this book. While I would prefer to write on a larger page than folded A5, portability seems to be more important at present.

A project journal

A project journal accompanies a project. The project could be moving house, academic research, the development of a creative work – anything in work or personal life that is a distinct event. The example used to illustrate the project journal is the journal that accompanied the writing of this book. Its origins were in notes (about learning journals) that began to accumulate around the time that the publishing proposal for the book was submitted. The notes were on A5 paper for portability and they were ring-bound. A reflective journal section started – it seemed to start itself up without prompting! Often the thinking was done in a period of physical exercise at the end of an evening of writing. From this reflective section, an idea of chapter topics emerged and sooner or later, within a new set of page dividers, material began to find its way from the general section into the chapters – sort of finding its way to its 'home'.

Reading of literature occurred alongside these journal activities and a coding evolved that enabled cross referencing. Ideas in the journal, however, were kept in a separate place from notes about other people's work.

In terms of the project notebook becoming a 'true' learning journal, the crucial decision was to make dated entries of reflection on the progress of the project. I did not record in the journal section every day, but it became the location for comments and for 'thinking on paper' about the progress of the book. Miller (1979) talks about the value of journals in enhancement of creativity because the passage of the thoughts is recorded so that the mind is clear to move on to other thoughts, while a record of the 'train' of thinking is retained. My experience is in accordance with her comment.

Although this was not a first book, the journal-writing process enabled there to be more consolidation of learning about the management of information and the whole book-writing process through the process of thinking on paper in one place. Thinking would otherwise have been in my head (with attendant concerns about the quality and reliability of memory) or on a series of scrap sheets consigned to the bin as soon as I had passed through that stage. For the writer, a project journal accompanies any project – whether work or non-work.

A journal in a professional development Master's programme (Morrison, 1996)

Various references have been made to Morrison's use of journal-writing in earlier chapters (1990, 1996). Morrison's work is interesting because it is rooted in theoretical ideas, promotes personal, professional and academic development and has a particular role in the course that he describes. The journal is employed in the context of a modular Master's degree in education. One of its roles is to support reflective practice over the period of study, 'developing in students, the ability to be self-monitoring, self-directive and professionally autonomous'. This has particular relevance in the potentially fragmented learning environment of a modular programme.

The development of reflective practice in Morrison's work is based on two models of reflection. The first, which he equates with Schön's reflection-in and reflection-on practice, concerns short-term matters such as specific events, rather than long-term issues of personal relationship to society (Schön, 1983). The long-term issues for reflection are the subject matter of the second model. The concerns of the second model relate to a person's state in a social setting, issues of power and empowerment with the aim as emancipation. Students are introduced to these models in the context of their journal activities. In terms of the subject matter of the first model, they are asked to reflect in a day-to-day manner on their programme, on their study habits, on their reading, on significant events, decisions, insights and the views that they hold. They are also invited to consider the progression and development in their knowledge, practice, attitudes, understanding and so on. This reflection is supported by banks of questions.

The second model of reflective practice is based on the work of Prawat (1991). Students are invited to consider developments in the functioning that underlies personal power – their 'voice', their view of themselves in their settings and their knowledge of and relationships to the power in those settings.

The journals are not themselves assessed and they were an early example of the technique of assessment now favoured by the writer – the development of a reflective commentary that cites from the journal, but in which the journal itself is not assessed. The students can then learn more from their writing.

Thinkpoint

Progoff talks about difficulties in getting started in writing:

> Sometimes when we set out to write these elaborations of our interior experience, we find it difficult to get started. Nothing comes . . . 'Nothing is here', we think. But we should not make that judgment about ourselves. If we are accustomed to the psychological jargon of modern times, we may also be drawn to make a quick diagnosis of ourselves, saying 'I am blocked'. But that is probably not the actual problem. More likely it is simply the operational difficulty of being unable to set the process into motion. With so many thoughts, partial beliefs and interior events from which to choose, we are not able to pick one on which to focus and begin. The difficulty lies in not having a starting point, for without a starting point, we cannot begin.
>
> (Progoff, 1980: 115)

Chapter 13

Activities to enhance learning from journals

Introduction

Activities such as those that are suggested in this chapter may be part of the structure of a journal or they may be offered to learners to use – if they wish. They are offered, therefore, somewhat in the same spirit as the 'tools' offered by Rainer (1978: Chapter 6), though there are many more on offer here. We have suggested in earlier chapters that it can be useful to consider the development of journal work in two phases – the first stage of helping writers to write in a basically reflective manner, and later enabling them to write at a deeper level. It is useful to have this structure in mind when working with activities so that the manner in which the activity is introduced can be slanted towards the appropriate level of work or purpose for setting the activity.

Learners will often find activities or exercises particularly helpful when they first start to write because the nature of an activity may lead them into reflecting when they are not initially confident in this form of working. An activity can help to vary the patterns of reflection. It can 'trip' writers into useful confrontations with issues that they have consciously avoided in free writing. In this sense, activities can deepen reflective activity.

While 'writing' is the word mostly used in this chapter, other forms of representation such as drawing may be used – and on the basis that different learning can emerge from the use of different forms of representation, there may be surprise, or unexpected learning may result.

The activities are organized in eight groups on the basis of broad similarity, but many could fit into other sections. In order to provide an accessible resource for those using journals, we have sometimes repeated journal activities in this chapter from earlier in the book. There are more examples of reflective learning activities in Moon (2004a).

Activities to encourage reflective writing

There are several exercises in the Resources section (Resources 3 to 5) that can help learners to get started with reflective writing. These are supported by Resource 2, A generic framework for reflective writing, and instructions (Resource 1).

Take a theme

Lindberg (1955) describes wandering along the seashore and finding shells and the using the shell as a means of moving into reflection on her life. She would describe the shell and, from her description, would move into her journal entry. For example, a whelk shell that housed a whelk and latterly a hermit crab enabled her to reflect on her need for shelter and what shelter meant to her in a psychological and physical sense. An object can focus attention and provide a starting point. It can inspire the writer to work with metaphor (see also Schneider and Killick, 1998).

Use questions

A number of examples of journal-writing systems have been introduced in this book where questions have been used to generate reflection. Sometimes the questions have been developed into a framework (e.g. Johns, 1994) which takes learners through a sequence of reflecting according to the requirements of the programme. Johns uses questions to guide reflection on an event or action involving the writer, in this case in nursing practice, and similarly Smyth's framework (1989) encourages reflection ultimately on power and politics of self in a social setting. Questions help learners to get started in reflecting or to deepen their reflection. They may be used in the early stages of journal-writing and learners can then be encouraged to be self-guided when they are ready. A well-posed question can lead reluctant writers into reflective activity before they realize that they are fulfilling the requirement of journal-writing. A useful and wide-ranging question for students on a course is: 'At this moment, how are you feeling about being a (discipline/subject) student?' (Hahnemann, 1986). Paul (1990) and Morgan and Saxon (1991) also provide some useful principles for questioning.

Generate questions

An intermediate stage between the use of pre-posed questions and unstructured writing is to ask learners to develop their own questions – either for themselves or for each other. Hahnemann (1986) suggests that before a class discussion on a topic, students are asked to write questions about the topic in their journals. A discussion is then held on the topic, and presumably students might be asked to reflect on the discussion afterwards.

Footprints

Footprints is a development of the Steppingstones activity developed by Progoff (1975). It is particularly useful for generating material on which to reflect and write, or for exploring an idea. On a particular topic, learners are asked to list around seven experiences (memories) of the topic in strict chronological order – from birth towards the present time. Examples of topics that could be used are 'experiences of learning' or 'the idea of "home", or 'feeling sorry for others'. As the list is written, it is likely that other memories that belong previously in the sequence will arise. These are used in a second list, and again are located in chronological sequence. A series of lists can be generated that usually surprise the learner in their extent, particularly where the initial reaction of the learner is 'I don't remember much about that'. It is also interesting to note that on different days, the same person is likely to write different lists. This suggests that psychological context of the listing process is influential in the listing process. The lists can be retained in the journal, and learners invited to reflect further on, for example, 'the item that surprised you', or 'the item that seems most relevant to your current experiences'. A development of the original listing activity of Progoff can greatly enhance the value of the process. The writers join each other in a group and each, in turn, picks one item out of her list and shares it. The open choice of items ensures that participants can feel safe. This process of sharing tends to be very enjoyable, with laughter usually arising. The exercise can be very useful for the purpose of bonding groups or helping new students to get to know each other. After a suitable period, the participants are asked to go back to their listing and write more lists. It is likely that the sharing of ideas with others will have triggered memories that they would not otherwise have considered. Later they can be asked to pick items as topics for reflective writing in journals.

Concept mapping or graphic representations of ideas

The material in a journal does not need to be written. Graphic techniques can generate new ways of seeing things that can then be explored further in writing. A concept map encapsulates an idea and the themes radiate from the main idea and subdivide hierarchically (Moon, 1999a). Buzan (1993) and Deshler (1990) elaborate on this. The technique can be used individually or in small groups to generate thought that can then be the subject of writing. Several people can make separate maps on a topic and then can compare them. There can then be reflective writing on the differences between the maps of different people. Concept mapping can demonstrate conceptual differences that underpin learning. Hadwin and Winne (1996) review studies of concept mapping as a study strategy per se.

Free-flow writing

In 1973, Elbow suggested that a good means of freeing the style and thoughts of writers is to let writing free-flow on a topic, not correcting or criticizing it for a period of time (e.g. ten minutes). He describes this process of writing as being like a sea voyage. 'For the sea voyage you are trying to lose sight of land – the place you began . . . In coming to a new land you develop a new conception of what you are writing about.'

Elbow's idea was incorporated into a technique called 'teacher journal' by Yinger (1985). Learners write in 'free-flow' for around ten minutes. If they run out of ideas, they are asked to write about how it feels to have run out of ideas. They then reread and reflect on what they have written, then dialogue with another about the experience in a manner similar to co-counselling (see p. 151). It would seem appropriate then to ask them to reflect and write again.

'Take a sentence'

Hahnemann (1986) asks her students to 'take one sentence from your readings that sparked your interest and write on its meaning'.

Reflecting on own writing

It may be useful to distinguish between reflection on the learning that emerges from one's writing, reflection on the process of writing in a journal and using a reread to generate ideas for further reflection. In more formal terms, any of these outcomes can be encouraged by use of a double entry technique where one side of the page is for descriptive writing and the other is for further reflections on that writing.

Show learners your journal (as their teacher), or the successful journals of others

Sharing the content of journals has a generally facilitatory effect on writing. Those new to journal-writing may welcome the opportunity to look at journals that have been written for a while. They may be shown by the writers who can give peer support, or they may be shown anonymous journals that exemplify good practice. Often those best in a position to guide new journal writers is a group of learners who have been writing journals over a period of time.

Write day-notes

Give learners small notepads or pads of stick-on paper ('yellow stickies') and ask them to fill in a note on what they are doing or thinking about on a regular basis for a couple of days, writing, for example, once every hour. This will provide material for reflection later.

Learning about and managing one's own behaviour

Studying aspects of one's own behaviour

Joanna Field (1952) wanted to learn more about her own behaviour. A simple example of the manner in which she learned more was to note at the end of each day what had made her happy during the day. This might be a moment, a person or an object. In a similar way, other life experiences can provide a focus for writing, but the regular feature of Field's recording allows an observation of pattern over a period of time. Regular recording of other experiences is suggested by Miller (1979). They might be peak experiences and observations of hang-ups.

Period log

This is, again, one of Progoff's journal activities, which is mentioned in the example in Chapter 12. It is based on an observation that one's life does not simply flow in a smooth and unchanging path, but, over periods of time, has one theme or dominant feeling which then changes. The period log records the characteristics of a period of time. Most frequently it will be the period of time most recent to the present, and the period will have stretched back as far as the dominant theme or feeling stretches back. From personal experience, this can be from a few days to a few months or longer. The period log gives a sense of the flow of life and it sets a useful context for the other aspects of journal-writing, whether they are for personal or formal educational reasons.

Sub-personalities

While the previous activity provided a longitudinal view of life, in a sense this one provides a cross-section. Miller (1979) suggests that journal-writing is a useful means of exploring and identifying one's sub-personalities, perhaps providing them with names and noting when they arise. Hunt (1987) also considers the study of sub-personalities. He suggests a method of exploration by use of personally-guided imagery.

Focusing the nature of reflection on an experience

The experience could be a weekend away in a new place and the reflection could be guided by the personal question 'what did I learn from the weekend?' It is interesting to question oneself very soon after the event, a day or two later, and later again, and then a few weeks later. What happens to the nature of memory over time? Following this process can be very interesting.

Dialogues

A number of writers mention the use of dialogues, but Progoff's approach is more sophisticated. Dialogues are like scripts for a play in which the writer 'converses' with another. In Progoff's approach, the 'other' might be a person, a part of oneself, a spiritual leader or mentor, an object, an event, a project, or anything or anyone with whom there is 'work' to be done. A helpful example might be some task to which one cannot get around. The dialogue could then explore the blocks. The writing often starts with a greeting to the other and a maybe a statement of the issue that is to be the subject matter of the dialogue. The technique is simply to write for oneself and wait 'to see' what the other will say back, recording it then, uncritically. When the writer has used this exercise with a group, it can be interesting to ask if anyone has any new insights. Not infrequently one or two participants will say that they have solved a problem that has been bothering them for a while.

In the context of this section, dialogues may be with oneself or with parts of oneself, or, perhaps, with a mentor or a real or imaginary spiritual guide.

Different perspectives

An incident is picked by the journal writers, and it is examined for the various perspectives that could be taken on it. The following are examples: in a classroom, one child may have quarrelled with another; in a hospital, a patient seems constantly to be unhappy with her situation and argues about decisions made about her treatment. In the first example, there may be the point of view of the teacher, the first child, the other child, other children who observed; and then there might be an object over which the children quarrelled – a book or a pencil, for example. There might be a clock on the wall that is showing the time creeping towards the end of the lesson – and so on. The reflective writing carries accounts of all of these elements, including the inanimate objects (e.g. 'I am a pencil. I thought I belonged to Carl but for some reason Tom has decided that I belong to him. Maybe he admires me . . .'). This is a creative activity that can, like the dialogues exercise (see above), bring surprising new perspectives to a situation.

Haiku

Haiku is a three-line poetic form with 17 syllables with five, seven and five on respective lines. Hunt (1987) suggests that the method of condensing character-istics of oneself or one's behaviour into such form is a useful method of self-exploration.

Recording of activity

This exercise returns to more concrete activity, but it produces valuable data for further reflection. The exercise consists of logging one's behaviour or thoughts at regular spaces of time, using an alarm to mark the time. A particularly useful version of this activity for generating discussion if several people have pursued it, is to record one's thoughts periodically thoughout a lecture or class.

Currere

This is technique that is mentioned by Pinar (1975) and several writers who interpret Pinar's work (e.g. Grumet, 1987; Miller, 1987). Pinar originally developed the exercise in the context of work on the nature of the curriculum in schools, but it has potential for other situations. In essence, the same topic for reflection is related initially in the present, and then with reference to its past, and a third section of writing anticipates the future. Grumet suggests that 'multiple accounts splinter the dogmatism of a single tale. If they undermine the authority of the teller, they also free her from being captured by the reflection provided in a single narrative.'

Autobiographical writing

There are many references to autobiographical writing in relation to journals and in other 'one-off' accounts, particularly in the teacher education literature. The development of autobiography can be a focus of attention in journal-writing, and rather than consist just of memories, can utilize activities such as those that are described in these chapters, such as currere, footprints, dialogues and so on.

Rehearsal

A helpful means of managing difficult or anxiety-provoking events such as conflict with another, examinations or driving tests is to rehearse them in advance. While they can be rehearsed in imagination, greater focus maybe obtained by writing them out. This might take the course of a dialogue or an account of the anticipated event with the writers seeing themselves successfully managing the situation. Going through the account several times and thinking about it is likely to facilitate the eventual enactment of the event for the writer.

Writing letters that are not to be sent

Again, several writers mention this technique (e.g. Rainer, 1978; Cooper, 1991). Like rehearsal, above, this is a method that can help with the management of personal behaviour. This might be particularly the case if the content is cathartic in nature.

Life decisions and the ways that were not followed

Progoff (1975) calls this work 'intersections'. Decisions may have implied the taking of one path in life and the rejection of another or others. Progoff suggests that sometimes there is still 'energy' left in the path(s) not taken and the course that events might have taken can be worthy of exploration. This is a kind of 'what if' exercise – and well worth while.

Metacognitive activities

Reflect on the act of journal-writing

Asking learners to reflect on the act of journal-writing can be useful in the manner that any act of metacognition appears to facilitate learning. It can be useful also as a means of unblocking writing if learners say that they do not know what to write – or it can be used as a 'filler' activity if there is a set period for journal-writing.

Self-assessment of own learning journal

If journals are to be assessed in a formal learning situation, asking learners to assess their own journals is another means of encouraging reflection on the act of writing a journal. The value of the exercise will be increased greatly if the development of assessment criteria is a collaborative activity between tutors and learners.

Reflecting on the process of writing an essay/report/other academic writing

An essay (or other piece of writing) is copied and put into the journal (if feasible). The journal writer then reflects on the process of writing the essay both in terms of the quality of the outcome, and the process of writing it. What thoughts, for example, came first and how were they developed?

Learners choose their own style of reflective writing

Setting a journal-writing task for learners is not always easy. There are many reasons that learners may find for arguing against the task. If there are difficulties, it may be worth turning the task initially into one of designing a format for ongoing recording and reflection that the learners then maintain (Stephani, 1999). The task may involve thought about the aims and purpose and outcomes of the writing – and the work may not, in the end, be called a journal.

Observations of personal learning through language

Parker and Goodkin (1987) describe a method of focusing on the manner in which the contribution of personal language to learning is explored by teaching students. They are asked to devote one journal entry per week to a description of an occasion when they have used language to learn something on their course. At the end of the year, they select four or five of these entries and write a short 'informal' paper on 'what they think they have learned about thinking and learning from this process' (Parker and Goodkin, 1987: 48).

Questions that focus on personal experiences of learning

An easy way to help learners to reflect on their own processes is to provide sets of questions that lead them towards reflection. The following set is an example:

- What are the characteristics of an interested and motivated learner?
- What are the characteristics of a non-motivated learner?

- Where do you stand? How do you fit these models?
- When have you been really involved in learning something?
- When have you found learning really difficult?
- What does the difference tell you about yourself?

The learners could decide their own questions or develop similar questions for each other.

Reflection on the process and results of a study skills (or other psychologically-based) questionnaire

The use of a questionnaire or scaling of some attribute can provide useful material for metacognitive reflection.

The process of learning in a class

A lecture or class is recorded. Elements of the material are played back to learners and they are asked to record what was in their minds at the time. The reports may be about the learning process or the content of the material. The outcome for a whole class may yield interesting material for teacher and students about the processes of teaching and learning.

Reflection on an interesting aspect of learning

Learners are asked to go over lecture notes or material from reading and mark the part that is of most interest to them and write about the reasons for that interest.

Learning from a negative emotional event

This activity can provide much useful information about the personal processes of reflecting and the role of emotion in the process. When an emotional event has occurred – something that has caused upset and in which others are involved, the journal writer writes a piece about the event as soon after it has occurred as possible, and then another account at a later stage (e.g. the next day), and one on the following day and then another a week later and then a week after that. It is very interesting to see how the feeling change at different time gaps . . . and it is interesting to think how this affects the writing of usual entries in a journal.

Consulting inner wisdom

A dialogue technique (see p.145) is set up between the learner and a 'wisdom figure'. The figure may be an imagined real person (a mentor) or a completely imaginary person or figure. The dialogue is about the writer's methods of study and learning, with advice being offered. This is similar to an example given by Cowan (1998b: 68–9).

Focus on one aspect of behaviour

Learners could be asked to focus on one aspect of their characters (e.g. shyness) and to explore it in as many ways as they can think of – sometimes just working alone, and sometimes working with others or reference materials.

Non-verbal methods for working in a journal

Doodle

Doodle. What words come up? What thoughts does the doodle draw from within you?

Draw an image

Progoff uses the drawing of images to facilitate reflection or to summarize a session of reflection. The image may be meaningful like a metaphor, or a graphic construction from the mind of the learner. Similar to this is to ask learners to summarize a lecture or area of knowledge, or a project, in an image in their journals. There may be writing to accompany the image. A variation on this is to engage in free drawing (as Milner, 1957).

The road map of life

This may be a useful activity with which to introduce journal-writing. The passage through life is depicted as a road over a map, like a route. The 'going' may be easy and comfortable (perhaps through beautiful countryside) or rough and bumpy (through steep mountains). There may equally be dark or light, open or closed areas of life. The means of depiction are unlimited. The exercise is probably better done initially on a large piece of paper which maybe reduced to fit into a journal, or which is treated as a resource to inspire writing. Like many activities, the map drawn on one day may be completely different on the next day; and the difference probably says something about the occasion of the activity. I did this exercise in the context of educational work with prisoners. While for most people the lines fade through the present into the future, the line for some of the prisoners came to an abrupt halt at the moment of their sentencing.

Holly (1991) suggests a similar activity, which she calls 'timelines', in which life is divided up into sections along a line (e.g. young childhood, adolescence etc.). Key words that relate to the sections and further exploration by way of photographs and other artefacts may be consulted in order to clarify the events.

Dreams

Recording dreams may help to elucidate concerns or issues in life or learning. There are many different books on the interpretation of dreams on the market, and many different methods of interpretation (e.g. Shohet, 1985). From personal experience, one of the most interesting is the Gestalt method in which an imaginary account of its role in the dream is written for each element of the dream (objects, abstract ideas and places as well as people). When worked out in this way, some elements of a dream may seem to be more significant to the dreamer's current concerns.

Twilight imagery

From personal experience and despite what dream books tell us, dreams cannot always be relied on to appear. Twilight imagery is a term developed by Progoff for the imagery that can spontaneously appear in a relaxed state which Progoff describes to be 'between waking and sleeping' (1975: 77). The imagery is, he suggests, representational or symbolic. The significance of images is that 'we do not consciously or deliberately put these perceptions there. We, ourselves, do not determine what they shall be' (1975: 78). They do, however, seem to be encouraged to flow if we take interest in observing them and recording them. In the section on journals to support creativity (Chapter 6), I described the appearance of a 'bear mouse' creature in my twilight imagery, and its importance to me.

Rainer suggests another version of twilight imagery. She suggests that the writer starts with an image, relaxes and 'watches' to see what happens.

Draw yourself or a project as a tree

A tree can be tall, strong, twisted, leafy, shady, growing in fertile or arid soil . . . There are many words that allow human characteristics to be projected onto the image of a tree and the exercise of projection can generate a useful summary and facilitate unexpected learning.

Cartoons

Regular journal writers could be asked to depict some entries in cartoons and other graphic forms and to reflect on how this is different.

Working with others on journal activities

In this section, we assume that the material is worked on in pairs or groups. The material may have arisen either from journals or as an outcome of the group/paired work. 'Footprints' is an example of an activity which involves working with others.

Co-counselling

The model of co-counselling is based on the work of Jakins (1970) and Evison and Horobin (1983), and both of these manuals contain activities within co-counselling. Co-counselling is a situation in which usually two participants work together in such a way that first one is listener/counsellor and the other talks, and then for the same length of time the situation is reversed. The 'talker' 'owns' the time, using it to explore an issue of his or her choice or one allocated in a formal situation. The talker may or may not want the listener to ask helpful questions or facilitate the process. Within the context of journal-writing, it is likely that the issue will be one that has arisen in the writing process. After the session, the new learning can be recorded.

Critical friends

The system of 'critical friends' is similar to co-counselling, although it may not need to occur in pairs. The difference is in the role of the listener who more actively prompts the talker in the manner in which he or she explores the issue in hand, asking questions that promote deeper reflection, and prevent avoidance of difficult issues.

Joint work on autobiographical material

This is a manner in which learners can help each other to write autobiographical material. One of a pair talks about his or her autobiography and the other prompts, questions and comments in order to work towards 'truths' and material that is useful to the present. The talker writes up the session in draft, and shows it the other who may question further. They work together to form material that is as accurate and helpful to present agendas as possible.

Authoring for another

Learners write entries as if they were seeing an event through the eyes of another (known) person. They discuss the outcomes and how they differ from their own accounts.

Development of concept maps

Several learners develop concept maps (see p. 143) on a topic that they have chosen or that has been given. They then share their maps and discuss the differences in perception of the topic. This is a means of emphasizing the differences in perceptions of the same activity or concept.

Dialogue journals

The literature on dialogue journals dates back a number of years. Early examples tend to emanate from primary school classrooms where pupils were asked to write comments about their classroom activities (thoughts, feelings, observations . . .) to which the teacher then individually responded. Subsequent examples involved lecturers and students (Staton, 1988) or students working together, or researchers working in collaborative inquiry (e.g. Roderick and Berman, 1984). Examples of literature on dialogue journals are given in Staton *et al.* (1988). The disadvantage of such a method can often be the time it takes for transmission and response, and modern versions of email discussions can overcome this.

Activities in journals used to support other learning

Improving the learning from creative processes

There are many situations in formal education where a physical object is the outcome of work and the object itself is the subject of assessment. Not only is the process of learning to create the object neglected in assessment terms, but there is a loss of opportunity to reflect on and during the process and to learn from this (Davies, 1998). Journals can play a valuable part in the creative process either to enable assessment to be made of the process, or to enhance learning.

Quick think

Learners are given a contentious topic relevant to their discipline. They are asked to discuss it for five minutes. Afterwards they are asked to reflect on the discussion. Words which may have variable definitions or 'what if?' topics are good subject matter for this exercise.

Use journals to enhance learning within the class

There are many ways in which journal-writing can enhance classroom learning, both by consolidating and demanding active learning and by providing a change of pace. Some of the suggestions below come from an extract on the internet edited by Jacobson (nd):

A question is displayed for learners when they come into the class. They spend five minutes on it in their journals. The question might initiate thinking about the subject matter of the session.

There is time for learners to write a summary of a class at the end of the session, or to note issues, or the most significant factors that they have learned (etc.).

Learners are given a break during a lecture to write a response to a question, to note issues that they least understand, or to summarize or develop thoughts.

A similar break is posited in a discussion session or a seminar.

Journals used alongside problem solving

Perhaps one of the most useful observations about the use of journals is that writing about the solving of a problem improves the process of problem solving

(Jacobson, nd; Selfe and Arbabi, 1986; Cowan, 1998b; and others). Learners write or talk about their processes of problem solving rather than following the process 'in their heads'. They seem better able to solve the problem at hand and to learn the process for a later problem.

Relating theory and practice

A number of writers (e.g. Hettich, 1976; Wagenaar, 1984; Fulwiler, 1986) use journals with their students to encourage the making of connections between the classroom theory and practical and real-world situations. They ask them to seek out examples of the classroom ideas in everyday life and to write them up in the journal.

Taking a wider picture on field-notes

Field-notes can be strictly scientific only or there may also be a section that is a means of recording personal feelings along with the observations. This seems to enable learners to 'see' and understand better the subject of their observation (Fulwiler, 1986). It probably aids their memories as well.

'What if?' questions

These may be part of a 'quick think' session (above) or an activity alone. 'What if?' questions stretch thought and imagination into areas not normally encountered.

Dialogue with works

This is another of Progoff's dialogue sections – and it is particularly appropriate for working with learners on topics in their disciplines (see p. 145). The dialogue might be with, for example, a theory, an object of art, a building in engineering, a project in scientific subjects, a planet, or a novel.

Select areas of confusion

Learners are encouraged to seek out and explore areas of work in which they are confused or uncertain. An atmosphere of trust enables learners to admit their difficulties (Mayher et al., 1983).

Activities to support reflective practice

A means of learning to reflect on practice

Neary (1998) introduces the notion of reflection on practice to groups of students early in their course by asking them to give a short and relevant presentation and to write a reflective account of their performance in their journals.

Relating one's own learning to that of others

Exploring one's own attitudes towards something or exploring one's processes of performing in some way can be reflectively compared with observations of the equivalent in others. Subject matter might be one's attitude towards authority in a particular and relevant situation.

Critical incident analysis

Critical incident analysis is often seen as a technique on its own that encourages reflective practice but within the context of a journal it is also a useful activity (Ghaye and Lillyman, 1997). A critical incident itself can be just an ordinary incident or one about which there is a special characteristic. In effect it is an incident that is selected for analysis with the expectation that learning from experience will result. The incident is described and then subjected to 'why questions' and other forms of deeper analysis in order to get at the unquestioned aspects of the event and in order to learn from them.

Situations in practice

Learners write about a situation that went well and one that went badly during the day/week. Adding two dimensions to writing with an element of contrast sets up a tension and leads to questions which can be brought to bear on the ensuing reflection.

Portraits

Working out relationships with others plays a large part in most practice situations. Rainer (1978) suggests the development of 'portraits' as an activity that enables the writer to gain a picture of another that is separated from the other's role in relation to the writer. Sometimes there is dislike for the person because he or she has something that is a problem similar to one within the writer him/herself. Issues that concern the relationship with others can be seen in a more objective light. The portrait is simply a written description of the person, but not the relationship.

Activities to deepen reflection and the learning from reflective processes

The series of exercises in the Resources section are designed to deepen reflective writing (Resources 3, 4, 5). They are supported by Resource 2: A generic framework for reflective writing. Full instructions are given in that section.

Metaphor

Many of the activities already mentioned involve the use of metaphor directly or indirectly. Richardson (1994) indicates how we tend to perpetuate 'worn-out metaphors' in writing. An example is the notion of theory as a building. She suggests that we should try considering theory as a tapestry or illness, and then notice the difference it makes to our perception. One way of working with metaphor in a journal is to highlight metaphors that we do use and examine in further entries how they affect the manner in which we view the matter. A progression from that stage is to try allocating new metaphors and determine the effect on perceptions.

Another use of metaphor is illustrated in part in a paper by Reid and Leigh (1998). As a means of assessment of an undergraduate module, students were asked to develop a three dimensional image as a means of promoting reflection on their learning about organizations. The step beyond the construction that makes this a good journal activity is the reflection on how the construction relates to the learning.

Altered points of view

The same event perceived by different people or from the viewpoint of different life stages of the same person (Rainer, 1978) or by sub-personalities (see p. 145) can seem very different. By enacting the different viewpoints about an indentified issue in the form of imaginary dialogues, it may be possible to attain a deeper and broader understanding of it. Weil (1996), for example, describes how her research on educational experiences was enriched considerably through her 'giving voice' to the different elements of her role as a researcher.

SWOT analysis

In some ways the use of a SWOT analysis is similar to the activity above in focusing on different groupings of factors that are a part of the same whole. A SWOT analysis is a review in terms first of strengths, then of weaknesses, then of the opportunities and lastly of threats to the possibility of change. The review might focus on a person and his or her capacities, an event, a project, a situation, a system – anything. A reflective overview of the analysis may demonstrate some surprises.

Repertory grid

The repertory grid is based on the work of Kelly (1955). Kelly's thesis is that people endeavour to make meaning from the elements of their environment in order to gain control over their lives. As humans, we develop a representational model of the world as a means of organization and the model is unique to an individual because it represents the sense he or she has made. The repertory grid technique elicits the meanings that we construct. In a very simple form it produces interesting data about the way in which we see the world. If the subject matter is the characteristics of people, three people are identified. On the basis of some characteristic, two are identified as similar and one different. The process is repeated with another three people and again a characteristic is identified that distinguishes two from one of them. The characteristics that have been selected represent elements of the construct of personhood for that individual. Eventually the selected characteristics will be repeated and this indicates that the extent of the construct is being reached. The repertory grid can be used for anything, not just people.

Write a poem

The writing of poetry can enable to emotional content of a topic to be more freely expressed. It can generate information about other aspects of the topic that later can be subject matter for more straightforward reflective writing.

Use of the absurd

When there is to be discussion on a problem or issue, ask learners to develop absurd comments or solutions if it is a problem and to write on them in journals. It is amazing how often these absurd comments/pieces of writing contain wisdom that would not otherwise be evident.

Multiple layers of reflection

This activity is an extension of the idea of double entry journals where initial descriptive writing is subjected to reflection at a later stage, with the reflective writing usually written in a column alongside the description, or on the opposite page. Multiple layer reflection is where there is another and perhaps yet another review of the initial description and its initial reflection, perhaps taking in increasingly broad ranges of entries and seeking patterns.

Thinkpoint

This extract is from the journal of Norman McCanch, a lighthouse keeper who recorded his experiences in many of the UK lighthouses while they were still manned. This was written when McCanch was manning the S. Bishop lighthouse off the Welsh coast.

> *July 26th* Last night, as the sun was going down, a single heron flapped slowly past the lighthouse and continued westwards until it was lost to sight. I was a bit surprised to see this purposeful expression of the migrating instinct in a bird I had never imagined to move across the Irish sea, but this morning two immatures followed the same ponderous course, followed only a few minutes later by a group of three . . . I spent the greater part of the day keeping an eye for signs of others moving west, or these intrepid individuals coming back . . . My vigilance produced no more herons . . .
>
> (McCanch, 1985: 106)

Resources

The material in this section may be freely photocopied, though it would be appreciated if the author's name and the source of the copy were included.

Resource 1   Instructions for exercises on the depth and quality of reflection (Resources 3, 4 and 5)

Resource 2   A generic framework for reflective writing. This framework supports and should be used alongside Resources 3, 4 and 5

Resource 3   Exercise: A GP's story

Resource 4   Exercise: The worrying tutorial

Resource 5   Exercise: The surprise at home

Resource 1

INSTRUCTIONS FOR EXERCISES ON THE DEPTH AND QUALITY OF REFLECTION (RESOURCES 3, 4 AND 5)

The aim of these exercises is to enable participants to see what reflective writing looks like, to recognize that reflection can vary in depth and that there is more potential for learning from deeper rather than superficial reflection. They are developed in response to the observation that students, who are asked to reflect, tend to reflect rather superficially. In the exercises there are three or four accounts of an incident. In each case someone is reflecting on the incident as she/he might if writing in a journal. The accounts are written at increasingly deeper levels of reflection. From the writer's experience of wide use of these exercises, the subject matter is not important. It is even disadvantageous to give an exercise with subject matter that relates to the discipline of the group because the group will then tend to put on their disciplinary hats and examine the issues from that point of view, rather than consider the qualify of the reflective learning.

The procedure for the exercise is described as a group process, though it can be used individually. The process works best when it has a facilitator, who is not engaged in the exercise. The exercises take around an hour and is best when the facilitator is very much in control of the situation. It is important, for example, that the pages of the exercise are not leafed through in advance other than as instructed and the exercise works better when people follow the instructions – in particular, not beginning the discussions until everyone has read the relevant account. The groups can be told that there are three or four accounts of an incident – according to the exercise selected, and that they will be reading them one after the other, with time after each session of reading for discussion about the reflective content of the account.

- The exercise is introduced as a means of helping the group to see what reflective writing looks like and to demonstrate that there are different depths in reflection and that deeper reflection probably equates with better learning.
- Small groups are formed (no more than six in each).
- The groups are told to turn to the first account and read it quietly to themselves, considering what features they think are reflective.
- When it is evident that most people have read the first account, the groups are invited to discuss the account and identify where and how it is reflective. They are given about five to seven minutes for each discussion session. They may need less time for the earlier accounts.
- After the discussion session, the participants are asked to read the next account in the sequence (and they are reminded not to turn pages beyond the account in hand).
- After the last account has been read and discussed, groups are asked to go back through all of the accounts and to identify features of the reflection that progressively change through the accounts. For example, the accounts change

from being 'story' to focusing on issues in the incident. In the later accounts there is more recognition that there are multiple perspectives, etc. The groups are asked to list (e.g. on flip chart paper) the ways in which the accounts 'deepen' – but not just to describe the qualities of each account.

- In a plenary, the groups share their lists (as above) and discuss the whole exercise. It is at this stage that the participants can be referred to the Generic Framework for Reflective Writing, which provides a general guide to features in deepening reflection. The accounts are not intended to accord directly with the stages described, but both are like continua running in parallel.

If the exercise is used with staff, and if they are likely to want to use it later with their own students, it is worth having spare copies available (participants tend to want to mark/underline text on their copies in this exercise).

(Material developed by Jenny Moon, Bournemouth University)

A GENERIC FRAMEWORK FOR REFLECTIVE WRITING

There are four 'levels' of depth of reflection described below. They do not necessarily accord directly with the accounts in exercises such as The Park, but provide a general guide.

Descriptive writing

This account is descriptive and it contains little reflection. It may tell a story but from one point of view at a time and generally one point at a time is made. Ideas tend to be linked by the sequence of the account/story rather than by meaning. The account describes what happened, sometimes mentioning past experiences, sometimes anticipating the future, but all in the context of an account of the event.

There may be references to emotional reactions but they are not explored and not related to behaviour.

The account may relate to ideas or external information, but these are not considered or questioned and the possible impact on behaviour or the meaning of events is not mentioned.

There is little attempt to focus on particular issues. Most points are made with similar weight.

The writing could hardly be deemed to be reflective at all. It could be a reasonably written account of an event that would serve as a basis on which reflection might start, though a good description that precedes reflective accounts will tend to be more focused and to signal points and issues for further reflection.

Descriptive account with some reflection

This is a descriptive account that signals points for reflection while not actually showing much reflection.

The basic account is descriptive in the manner of description above. There is little addition of ideas from outside the event, reference to alternative viewpoints or attitudes to others, comment and so on. However, the account is more than just a story. It is focused on the event as if there is a big question or there are questions to be asked and answered. Points on which reflection could occur are signalled.

There is recognition of the worth of further exploring but it does not go very far. In other words, asking the questions makes it more than a descriptive account, but the lack of attempt to respond to the questions means that there is little actual analysis of the events.

The questioning does begin to suggest a 'standing back from the event' in (usually) isolated areas of the account.

The account may mention emotional reactions, or be influenced by emotion. Any influence may be noted and possibly questioned.

There is a sense of recognition that this is an incident from which learning can be gained, but the reflection does not go sufficiently deep to enable the learning to begin to occur.

Reflective writing (1)

There is description but it is focused with particular aspects accentuated for reflective comment. There may be a sense that the material is being mulled over. It is no longer a straightforward account of an event, but it is definitely reflective.

There is evidence of external ideas or information and where this occurs, the material is subjected to reflection.

The account shows some analysis and there is recognition of the worth of exploring motives or reasons for behaviour.

Where relevant, there is willingness to be critical of the action of self or others. There is likely to be some self-questioning and willingness also to recognize the overall effect of the event on self. In other words, there is some 'standing back' from the event.

There is some effort to respond to questions posed.

There is recognition of any emotional content, a questioning of its role and influence and an attempt to consider its significance in shaping the views presented.

There may be recognition that things might look different from other perspectives, that views can change with time or the emotional state. The existence of several alternative points of view may be acknowledged but not analysed.

In other words, in a relatively limited way the account may recognize that frames of reference affect the manner in which we reflect at a given time but it does not deal with this in a way that links it effectively to issues about the quality of personal judgement.

Reflective writing (2)

Description now only serves the process of reflection, covering the issues for reflection and noting their context. There is clear evidence of standing back from an event and there is mulling over and engagement.

The account shows deep reflection and it incorporates a recognition that the frame of reference with which an event is viewed can change.

A metacognitive stance is taken (i.e. critical awareness of one's own processes of mental functioning, including reflection).

The account probably recognizes that events exist in a historical or social context that may influence a person's reaction to them. In other words, multiple persectives are noted.

Self-questioning is evident (an 'internal dialogue' is set up), deliberating between different views of personal behaviour and that of others.

The view and motives of others are taken into account and considered against those of the writer.

There is recognition of the role of emotion in shaping the ideas and recognition of the manner in which different emotional influences can frame the account in different ways.

There is recognition that prior experience and thoughts (own and other's) interact with the production of current behaviour.

There is observation that there is learning to be gained from the experience and points for learning are noted.

There is recognition that the personal frame of reference can change according to the emotional state in which it is written, the acquisition of new information, the review of ideas and the effect of time passing.

(Material developed by Jenny Moon, Bournemouth University)

A GP'S STORY

Account 1

Early January – it is always like that – cold outside, hot and airless inside and the post-Christmas ailments come pouring in. I had had a bad night. Our 17-year-old had gone out clubbing with her friends and phoned at 2.00 a.m., unable to find a taxi – would one of us come and get her. As soon as the phone was down, Julia, my wife, plausibly argued the case for staying in bed because of her teaching day the next day. (What about my long list in the surgery today?) I didn't argue – just got up and went. It was hard getting up in the morning and it was a particularly long list of the worried well, with coughs and colds and 'flu' being used to hide their family discords and boredoms with work. I'm cynical – OK.

I was getting towards the end when the door opened on Marissa. She came in – hunched shoulders, grey-faced as usual – and clutching her bag in that peculiar way. She is 30, but always manages to look twice her age. Our practice is well aware of Marissa and her aches and pains. I was a bit surprised to see her because she had not been on the list when I first saw it this morning so that meant that Trisha, our receptionist, must have squeezed her in. Trisha's expertise at judging who needs to be 'squeezed in' is usually accurate and would not tend to include the heartsinks like Marissa.

I welcomed Marissa in. She had a wrenched shoulder this time and she said that it had happened when she was lifting a bed in her mother's house. It was a slightly unusual one for Marissa. She was more of the tummy-ache and headache brigade. I had a quick look and prescribed painkillers. I typed the prescription and looked up, expecting the relieved look, but it was not there and she asked me if the painkillers would really take away the pain. I was a bit perplexed and I asked her why she had been moving furniture. She started to tell me how she had decided to move back to live with her mother. In my tired state at this end of the morning, I prompted questions about her family relationships and she seemed to open up. I felt I was doing the right thing – even felt noble about giving her the time on that morning, but I knew I was not very 'sharp' about it. I thought that just letting her talk for a few moments was probably helpful to her.

Marissa had been born long after the other children and felt as if she had been seen as a nuisance, particularly by her mother. But now she could not cope alone and was moving back in with this cold mother. I had got her talking and I brightened, thinking I was doing a good job. I wondered why I had not let this talk flow before. We ran out of time, and I asked her to come back to talk more. I was thinking that we might be able to get on top of these recurrent visits to the surgery.

I did actually feel better after seeing her. My attitude to my 'success' with her changed the next week. Marissa did come back – but not to me. She chose to come back when Geoff, the senior partner, was on. She was still complaining about the shoulder and she told Geoff that I had obviously thought that her shoulder was to do with her family – but it was not and she needed more than painkillers. Looking at the shoulder, Geoff agreed with her and referred her for physiotherapy. This little incident has perturbed me a bit. It stirred up my professional pride. I had thought I was doing a good job.

Account 2

There was a recent event that made me think a bit about the way I see patients and the manner in which I work with them. I'd had a short night and there were some bad feelings around at home. It was difficult to feel on top of the job and to cap it, it was also early January. We tend to get into the surgery lots of patients with the after-effects of the Christmas period then – the colds, the 'flu's and those who do not want to go back to work. All this makes me irritable when the lists of genuinely ill patients are almost too long to manage. I am not sure how much this generally bad start had to do with the event – how much has my own state to do with how I function?

So it was the end of this particularly long morning when Marissa walked in. Marissa had not been on the list that I had seen earlier and I was surprised that Trisha (the receptionist) had added her – since it is the 'genuinely' ill patients who are added once the list has been made up. Marissa is a regular with minor aches and pain. Sometimes there is just not time for these patients – but how do we solve that? I welcomed Marissa. She was pale and hunched as usual. She told me that she had a wrenched shoulder from when she had been moving a bed in her mother's house. I had a quick look: I had probably diagnosed a simple muscular sprain even before I examined her shoulder. I made out prescription for painkillers. When I looked up, she was still looking at me and asked if the painkillers would really take the pain away. I was surprised at her question – and clearly should have taken more note of it. Instead, I launched into a little bit of conversation, hoping to shift on to the next patient quite quickly. I asked her why she had been moving furniture and she started to tell me how she could not cope alone any more and had decided to move back in with this mother who did not seem to care for her. As she talked, I thought that she seemed to brighten up and I felt that I must be on a helpful track. I wonder now if I brightened up because I thought I was being helpful for this patient. We ran out of time and she agreed to come back the following week to discuss it all further. I was hoping after that to pass her on to the counsellor and we might be able to sort something out that would prevent the recurrent visits.

I felt better in myself after the session. It felt like one of those times when the professional work is going well. Trisha even commented that I looked brighter. 'Yes', I said, 'I did some good work this morning with Marissa.' I wished I had not said that.

Marissa did come back, but she came back at a time when Geoff, the senior partner, was on. She said to Geoff that I had been asking her all sorts of questions about her family and that what she wanted was help for her shoulder. She said that the painkillers were no good – and she had known that at the time I had prescribed them – hence, I suppose, the comment that she had made. Geoff had another look at her shoulder and was not happy about it. He referred her for physiotherapy. And then he told me all about the session with her and I felt very responsible for my mistake. I did not say anything to Geoff about how I had been feeling that morning.

It felt relevant, but perhaps I should be superhuman. When I look back on this incident, I can see that there are things that I can learn from it. There are all sorts of intersecting issues and feelings tangled up in there. Life is so difficult sometimes.

Account 3

A particular incident in the surgery has bothered me. It concerns Marissa, a 30-year-old woman who visits the surgery regularly for minor complaints (abdominal discomfort/headaches). She presented with a wrenched pain that was incurred when she was moving a bed in her mother's house. I diagnosed a muscular strain and prescribed painkillers. I suppose that I assumed that because it was Marissa, it was likely to be similar to her usual visits and that she may need little more than a placebo. She came back to the senior partner, Geoff, a few days later saying that I had not taken her shoulder seriously enough. He examined her and referred her for physiotherapy, as I can now see as appropriate management.

The event stirred up a lot of other things. The context was important. It was a January morning with the surgery full of worried well with 'flu's and the post-Christmas traumas. I came in tired and irritable because of family issues at home. Marissa was not on the list to start with. Trisha (our receptionist) added her because she judged that she needed to be seen that morning. Instead of taking note of Trisha's excellent judgement, I took this as a usual visit. This was a cue that I missed. Trisha knows Marissa and knows her behaviour when she books an appointment. She recognized this as different. This is an aspect of the teamwork that we aspire to in the practice.

Marissa came in and I did look at her shoulder – but I know that I had already made a judgement about it before I examined her. This was Marissa, looking, as usual, pale and hunched – and I saw any symptom as an expression of her state and nothing else. My look at the shoulder seemed an irrelevant act as I judged it then. I think about the many discussions of how easy it is to get misled by preconceptions and there was I doing just that. I can see that I should have taken the shoulder more seriously. Marissa, herself, asked if the painkillers were all she needed. What would it have taken for Marissa to have said to me that I was on the wrong track that day, and to have brought my attention back to her shoulder? I wonder if she knew that I was feeling 'off' that day. I suppose I did respond to Marissa's persisting discontent by launching into questions about her family situation – in particular her relationship with her mother and why she was going back to live there – things that later Marissa said were irrelevant.

When I stand back now and think of the event like a film, I can see how I was wrong-footed when Marissa questioned the initial prescription and did not seem any happier as a result of getting it. I just grabbed at the story she had given me. When she seemed willing to talk more about her family, I turned it to my favour – seeing myself as 'obviously' being helpful. That day, I think I needed to feel successful. If I am utterly cynical, I would say that I used Marissa's situation to alter my mood. But then again, I suppose, that in turn might have helped the patients whom I saw after her that day.

I need to think, too, about Geoff's role in this and about my relationships with him and the rest of the team. I am the most junior and I tend to look up to them. I suppose I want to impress them. I could talk this one over with Steve, one of the other partners, he might see it all differently.

Account 4

I write about an incident that continues to disturb me. I have gone over it several times and my perspectives seem to change on it – so I talked it over with Steve (one of the other partners) to see how he saw it. The incident concerns Marissa, a 30-year-old woman who visits the surgery frequently with various aches and pains (mostly tummyaches and headaches). The symptoms have never been serious, though she never looks well, nor does she seem happy. On this visit she presented with a wrenched shoulder which she said resulted from moving a bed. I did a brief examination and prescribed painkillers. There still seemed to be something bothering her so I engaged her in conversation about her family relationships (this arose from the circumstances of moving the bed). I thought she was responding well and we might be getting somewhere. Time ran out and I invited her to continue the conversation next week. I wanted to get her to a point where I could easily refer her to the practice counsellor. She agreed to come back – but came back to see Geoff, the senior partner, still complaining about the shoulder. He gave her a more detailed examination and referred her for physiotherapy. He told me that she said that I thought that her family was the problem when it really was her shoulder.

I can see now that the shoulder was a problem and I misconstrued the situation, engaging in the talk about her family. This was a multiple mistake. I did not pay attention to Trisha's judgement in adding Marissa to the list, I missed the shoulder problem itself when I examined it, but I also missed the cues that Marissa gave me when she was not happy with the prescription. But I was tired and out of sorts – not as sharp as I need to be when I am with patients. I am human, but I am a professional human and professionalism dictates that I should function well. I suppose that the problem was not so much that I missed one, or even two, cues – then I could have put things right. I missed all three at the same time.

I then headed off on the wrong track – getting into the discussion that I assumed was relevant about her family. I think of a consultation with our local GP when I was 14. I did not agree with his diagnosis about my foot – he just said I should come back in four weeks if it was not better. I did not say anything then, though I knew in myself that it needed treatment. I ended up in plaster for six weeks. There is a power thing there. Looking at it from Marissa's point of view, she may have known that I was on the wrong track, but she probably would not have been able to do anything about it because I am a doctor. Someone like Marissa would not question a doctor's judgement at the time. How often were principles like this drummed into us at medical school – and yet it seems so easy to forget them.

There is something more there too, though – this is what Steve suggested. That day, maybe I needed to feel helpful even more than usual – I needed more satisfaction from the situation, so I was looking for cues from Marissa that suggested that she was pleased with me. I had to make do with the cue that suggested that she was no longer unhappy and I suppose I made up the rest – thinking that the conversation about her family must be helpful. Maybe I can be more self-critical when I am in a better mood and less tired. Maybe I need less and can give more then.

It is possible, of course, that the conversation was not wrong in general, but wrong for that time. It may be helpful to her in the longer term – I just need to wait and handle the situation more mindfully when she comes back.

I can see that there are lots more issues in this – for example, I need to consider why I was so disturbed by the incident. I know I made a mistake, but I think if it had been Steve whom Marissa had consulted, I would not have been so bothered. It was worse because it was Geoff. Steve would have mentioned it and laughed. Once we have discounted serious symptoms it is not unusual to rely on patients returning quite quickly if they feel that a symptom is not disappearing in response to initial treatment. Geoff preached a bit and I responded by getting into my 'I am only junior' mode.

So what have I learnt?

- I am apt to see things differently when I am tired.
- I should pay attention to Trisha's judgements. She is the point of first contact and is pretty experienced in perceiving a patient's needs.
- I should be more aware about the power issues and how they silence patients. Maybe there are ways in which I can deal with this better. I will think on this.
- It was really useful talking the matter through with Steve. Hearing what I said to him enabled me to get it better into perspective and to see the issues in different ways.
- . . . Etc. (more issues listed).

(Material developed by Jenny Moon, Bournemouth University)

THE WORRYING TUTORIAL

Ian is 28. He is in the middle of the final year of a degree in biological sciences. He has worked in an agricultural laboratory prior to his degree programme and has embarked on the programme in order to take a post in agricultural research. Like many mature students, he has responsibilities at home that prove to be distractions to his degree work. He has just seen Pam, his tutor, for feedback on a recently marked essay.

Account I

I am gutted. I saw Pam this morning. She wanted to talk about my ecology essay. She was blunt. She said that I have not had any 'good' marks for work that I have done for the last year and a half – but none have been as near to failure as this one. She called this a 'hair's breadth pass' and she laid it on the line that I need to put in more effort all round or I will not be getting the degree that I need to work on research at Cummings. If I don't get that job, I could well end up with the same job that I did before and all this money and effort will have been pointless.

It seems that my essay was too descriptive and Pam tried to tell me what she meant by that. The title asked me to discuss the concepts of tolerance and limiting factors in relation to two named wild populations. I used Jencks and Parner's study of *abiniculus alba* and Cristom's study of *chyrups dipimus*. We covered the latter in a lecture and were given the reference for the other so I thought they were all right. Pam said that I should have found my own examples. She says that I write too factually. I need to make it clear that I realize that theories are not the same as facts. I need to think about how I use references. At this level I should question the data that I am working with – I should analyse and criticize it – not just accept it. She says that I'm good at assembling facts but that is not good enough now. Pam said that I should ask Tim if I can see some of his recent essays in order to get the idea and maybe I should go and see the study counsellor. I used to be good at essays. It seems that suddenly I am not.

I did really well in the first year of the degree. I felt that I knew most of the material that we covered – I had learnt it in my day-to-day work, though some-times I had to reinterpret it for the this academic context. Essays used just to flow out and I got good marks. I did do some reading and I would add a few references. I am not clear where those abilities have gone to. Suddenly I am not good any more. I suppose that some of it is to do with the baby. Pam and I did talk about how hard it is for me to study since Angie had the baby last year. Angie was ill over the pregnancy and after the birth. I was up in the nights and so tired and now I cannot concentrate at home because the baby is on her feet and all over everything. When I was trying to write the ecology essay she was teething and was not sleeping in the evenings. It is really hard being a student at this time in my life. The younger ones just don't know how easy they have got it.

I feel so gutted that I really don't know how I can go home at present. Angie still thinks that I am top of the class. I could not tell her. She has such faith in me – and I must get the new job in order to justify the hassle and expense of going back into education.

Account 2

Pam, my tutor, has talked with me about the essay I did for ecology and my progress in general. I have to face up to the fact that the mark was poor. If I do not do better, I will not get the research job at Cummings – and will be going back to the same job that I did before the degree and getting the new job was the whole point of doing the degree. I have felt so bad about this session with Pam and what it implies for me that I have not wanted to go home this evening. I know it is because I do not want to tell Angie that I am not as good at study as she thinks I am. She has such faith in me and I know that I am resistant to shaking that faith. However, I can see that I need to make some changes at home and until I talk to Angie, those changes will not make sense to her. What do I do or say?

Pam knows the difficulties that I had at home in the last year – in particular the distractions that occurred with the pregnancy and birth and with Angie's health. I suppose that my work began to deteriorate from around that time. I knew it was happening. Pam reminded me of several occasions when she told me that I should be doing some reading around the lectures but I somehow thought that I would get through and did not bother too much. I thought that a few poorer marks would not be a problem because I had done so well before and that really I did know how to write good essays.

Maybe I need to think about what Pam said about my essay. She says it is too descriptive and not analytical and discursive. She says that I am good at 'assembling facts' but that is not good enough for now and I should use my own examples – not those given in lectures. I need to think about what she means by that. I suppose that it means that I can write well but that is not well enough now and I need to be more original. What does she mean by analyse and discuss? She also says that I need to distinguish between theory and fact. I suppose that there is a difference that I need to consider and that may have something to do with the ways I use referencing that she also mentioned. It seems that I need to change the way in which I see the task of writing essays. I'll ask Tim how he writes such good essays. Pam says that Tim's essays are a good example. She also mentioned the study skills person, some books and coming back to her when I have thought about it.

So here I am, in the middle of my last year and in danger of not doing well enough to achieve what I must achieve for the future welfare of my family. What once seemed simple does not seem simple any more and it is all contorted by how well I did in the first year, and the frustrations (and joys, of course) of having a new baby. There is something about the image that Angie has of me as the great success story. Have I got to change that? All these things are floating around in there. I hope that they sort themselves out.

Account 3

I want to think about the tutorial I had with Pam. It was about my ecology essay and the very low marks for it. It was a seriously low mark. Pam also talked more generally about my lack of achievement. I noted down what she said about it, but it hurts to acknowledge it. Basically Pam says that the essay and my current prospects are both poor and she points out the increasing likelihood that I will not get a sufficiently good degree to get the research job at Cummings. It is the purpose of getting that job that brought me to university with all the sacrifices that has meant. When I look at the notes I wrote, my anxiety levels shoot up and I know I have to act. On previous occasions (not as heavy as this) I have just thought about it a bit and then I suppose I have gone back to the old assumptions that I would be all right because I am really a good student.

Where did those assumptions come from? I was well ahead in the first year and I had no problem in putting down material that was acceptable in essays. That might link up with what Pam said today about me being good at 'assembling facts'. Maybe that is what was wanted in the first year of the course and maybe she is really saying that doing that is not acceptable now. I am not totally clear from what Pam said what is wanted now – but it seems that most of my classmates do know. I will list the things that Pam said about my essay and work on them until I really understand what I need to do to write a good essay. Pam talked about things I could do. I must do them.

Now I start to think, things begin to link up. Pam and I talked about how disruptive last year was for my studies – with Angie being pregnant and ill, and with Meg's birth. Then, Pam was very sympathetic and even today I got into the 'poor me, how hard it is to be an adult student' stuff again. But then I am thinking that that attitude will not get me the degree and the job I want and I need to see it now as a convenient excuse. I did well in the first year because I knew the stuff, and then rested on my success when everything went haywire. I assumed that I could just re-engage – but I did not realize that the game had changed. What is asked for now is something different – not just the assembly of facts any more.

That brings me to why I am still in the library this evening and it is late and I have not gone home. I don't want to go home and tell Angie that I am not doing as well as she thinks. She assumes that I am still doing brilliantly – though last year she did question how I could be doing so well on so little work. I need a big shift in thinking – fast – and Angie is where I start. I need to tell her honestly about the tutorial, the feedback and my disappointment in myself. I am not the success that both of us assumed. I need her support so that I can get through this next six months and into the job and Angie's turn will come.

I list what I need to do apart from talking with Angie: I need to find out how to write a good essay at this stage in my degree. I need to find out what it means to 'discuss' and analyse and to sort out what a 'theory' is in ecology. I realize that I have never quite understood why we have theories about some things and we simply 'know' about other things. It seems that there is something different in ecology from the stuff that seemed 'factual' in the basic biology stuff. I need to think about these things and form them into clear questions so that I can find out what I need to know and how to put it on paper in an acceptable way. I think that the referencing will fall into place if I get these things sorted. Asking Tim may help only if I am clear about what I need to know. I will go back to Pam when I have done the thinking as well. Pam mentioned a couple of books and a website and the study skills person (make appointment tomorrow). There was also that research student I talked to in the bar the other night. I think I could talk more with him – but first I need to be focused about the information that I need.

(Material developed by Jenny Moon, Bournemouth University)

Resource 5

THE SURPRISE AT HOME

Emma is a student at the beginning of the third year of a degree in Geography. She is at a university a long way from home and has never come home unexpectedly before.

Account 1

I went home unexpectedly last weekend. I would never have thought of flying but it was incredibly cheap. It was Mum's birthday too and I thought it would be a nice surprise. I made a cake and took it. When I got home the surprise was on me – no, I should say it was a serious shock and I am still reeling from it. I remember walking up to the door, birthday cake, present and card in hand, ready to surprise them. I knocked instead of just letting myself in. I heard Jack barking and Tom, my 11-year-old brother called out to Jack from his bedroom. Then there was a scuffling and I saw the living-room curtain move. It was my Mum's face – but she looked different. I don't even think she took in that it was me. A few minutes later she came to the door – and she was different. I have never seen her wearing make-up like that and she had on a short dress with a low neckline. While she seemed genuinely pleased to see me in one sense, she was tense and jumpy but also giggly and several times said she wished I had let her know that I was coming. At that time I could not see why. I wondered why Dad did not come to the door though there was some sound in the background. Thank goodness Jack welcomed me as usual with his very waggy tail – and soon my brother was down in his pyjamas and hugging me. It was nice, but that was not his usual behaviour. Mum even said 'Come in', as if she was inviting a guest into the house. Then she said 'Come and meet my friend Jerry – he is an old friend who has just popped in'. I did not think he had 'just popped in' and I asked about Dad, 'Where is he?', and suddenly my mother seemed even more unsteady and I realized she had been drinking. My mother does not usually drink much. I had never seen her like this before. She seemed not to want to talk about Dad, saying in a clipped way that he was off on business. I know he is away a lot with his new job – but he would not be away on her birthday. Then the man called Jerry came out. I did not like him from the start. I felt as if something massive had happened to my family and that he was at the centre of it – and no-one had told me. We went into the living room. There were signs of a birthday – a mess of paper and chocolates and flowers – and a champagne bottle. It was not a family birthday-sort-of celebration – and Mum does not usually invite me to sit down . . .

I finally got to talk to my brother. His world was the rugby world cup at the moment. He said he'd seen Jerry a few times, especially when Dad was away and Jerry had been there a couple of mornings recently too. I think my brother knew things were different but he seemed to have swallowed the story of Jerry being an old friend who needed accommodation at present. I think he did know more and had shut it out.

Jerry was not there the next morning and Dad was apparently due back, but when he arrived there was a huge tension between Mum and Dad. It was really hard to communicate with either of them. There were one-word answers to any question and no-one seemed remotely interested in my life at Uni. But nothing was said about the situation and I did not know if Dad knew about Jerry. It was like my arrival was more than anyone wanted to cope with.

I am back now at Uni – still reeling on lots of levels – and very unsure about how to deal with it all.

Account 2

I went home unexpected last weekend, thinking I would surprise my mother because it was her birthday. It was me who was surprised. I sensed that there is something seriously wrong with the relationship between Mum and Dad and I think that a man called Jerry is involved. I don't know how much Dad knows and I don't know what to do – but I want to do something.

I got home and knocked at the door with the birthday cake in my hand and eventually Mum came out. She was surprised to see me, but not surprised with pleasure but with embarrassment. She was in a sexy dress with more make-up than usual and had been drinking. Soon a man came out. She introduced him as 'an old friend' who had just come round for a visit. When I went into the sitting room, there was a bit of a mess – paper and chocolates and champagne – it did not seem like a family celebration. My mother behaved differently. She was giggly but jumpy – not at all as I had expected. I felt hurt when she repeated several times that she wished I had let her know that I was coming. The whole point was to give her a birthday surprise. I did not sense that she was thinking about me at all.

I wondered where my father was on her birthday. I asked about him right in front of Jerry, but it felt as if I was saying the wrong thing. There was a brief silence and then I was told he was 'on business'. I was surprised again. I was beginning to guess what was going on, but was I right? No-one seemed to think I had a right to know.

My young brother was there. He was uneasy but really pleased to see me. It was a while before I could get to talk to him alone. On the surface he was 'matter-of-fact' – Jerry had been there a few times – sometimes in the morning too – and those times, Dad was away. I wanted to push my brother further, but I realized that he had to live with the situation and he was more or less coping at present. Was it fair to tell him my suspicions?

Jerry was not there the next morning. I did not do what seems now to have been appropriate – to tackle Mum about the situation. She just seemed so distant. Should I have challenged her? What rights do I have in this situation? Why didn't she talk to me? Dad was expected and I waited to see how things were. When he arrived, the tension between them was obvious. They bickered on and on and again I felt hurt that they seemed unable to recognize the effort I had put into coming home. I remember Sal (a friend at Uni) having a similar experience with her parents. She said that one of the worst things was the feeling that they lost interest in her and what she was doing in her life at the time. She felt she was set adrift and that was in addition to her worries about the stability of her family and the consequences of potential break-up.

So here I am, back at Uni and looking back on a traumatic weekend and thinking it all over again. There are all sorts of things floating around – emotions, hurt, worries about the future for me and my brother. Some of my initial reactions look different now. Have I have got it all wrong? Is my Mum having a little fling? Does that matter? Maybe my Dad is having an affair and that her fling is a reaction to his behaviour. Could I be making a huge mistake? I want to do something and yet I don't know what. What are my responsibilities here and to whom? Perhaps I should leave it for a few days and see how I feel then – though this worry is getting in the way of my work at Uni. I could try getting in touch with my brother to give him support, and I might get more information and then I can review what I should do.

Account 3

An incident happened, which has left me feeling very unsettled, wanting to take action, but unsure what to do and it is getting in the way of my work at Uni. I went home as a surprise for my mother's birthday. I do not normally go home like that, home being 300 miles away. I was looking forward to the family being surprised and pleased to see me. When I arrived, my mother had a 'visitor', Jerry. My Dad was away. According to my brother, Jerry has visited and apparently stayed the night several times when my Dad has been away. My mother seemed very embarrassed. She acted oddly, and looked different in dress and the amount of make-up. She had also been drinking. Jerry was gone the next morning and my Dad was due. Mum was more herself until Dad came and then the tension grew and they bickered more than I have heard before. I find it difficult to interpret the situation in any way other than as an affair, but I don't know for sure. My brother lives at home. He is 11. He did not say anything about my parents' relationship but I could see he was behaving a bit unusually. I felt he was coping and I don't want to unsettle him by asking difficult questions. I wonder if anyone else knows what is happening. Auntie Sue – my mother's sister – might know something and I have always got on well with her – or there is tackling my mother.

I try to separate out some of the parts of this. There is a factual side – what seems to be happening. I need to remember that my observations may not be well-founded. While it seems likely that my mother is involved in another relationship, the same may be true of my father. He was not there on her birthday. There will be two sides to the story whatever is happening – not just the side that I have seen. The ways in which it affects my brother and me are different too. We cannot help but be involved because they are our parents and we are part of the relationship between them. (I write that down and then wonder how they would see that. Maybe they would say that some of their relationship is between them only. Thinking that makes me feel even more unsettled.)

There is also the emotional side. I know that one set of feelings that are mine alone are about the welcome that I did not get on making the effort to go home. There is disappointment and a bit of anger that my parents could be so wrapped up in themselves. I suppose that those feelings will go in time and I know that the other things are bigger. I feel desperate if I think that my parents might separate or divorce. I know it is common and I don't suppose anyone ever thinks it will happen to them. If I felt neglected, my brother could feel the same – eventually a lot worse, and he will need my support very much.

Then there is the matter of what I should do. I don't want to ask Mum directly if she is having an affair with that Jerry – I feel a resistance to that in case I am wrong. Talking to Jules in my flat about her experience of parents breaking up has helped. Jules pointed out that even if things are not as they seem to be, it sounds as if something *is* going on. She is right – my parents were definitely not behaving normally. I am affected by it and my Uni work is suffering and therefore there is an issue. Jules thinks I should talk to my Mum and get it into the open. I suppose that I am looking for some facts to go on before I tackle her. I could just tell her I am very upset by what was happening when I visited – without being explicit. Then I will see what she comes out with and where it goes from there. That will help me to understand how to deal with it all. There may be an explanation that is less bad than it seems. That seems to be a useful strategy to start with. If when I talk with Mum, I have reason to continue being disrupted, I would ring Auntie Sue. Whether or not she knows, she will still help me and I need to get someone local to keep an eye on my brother and how he is managing.

(Material developed by Jenny Moon, Bournemouth University)

References

Alerby, E. and Elidottir, J. (2003) 'The sounds of silence: some remarks on the value of silence in the process of reflection in relation to teaching and learning', *Reflective Practice* **4**(1): 41–51.

Allport, G. (1942) *The Use of Personal Documents in Psychological Science*, New York: Social Science Research Council.

Alterio, M. (2004) 'Collaborative journaling as a professional development tool', *Journal of Further and Higher Education* **28**(3): 321–33.

Alterio, M. and McDrury, J. (2003) 'Collaborative learning using reflective storytelling', in N. Zepke, D. Nugent and L. Leach (eds) *Reflection to Transformation*, Palmerston North: Dunmore Press.

Ambrose, J. (1987) 'Music journals', in T. Fulwiler (ed.) *The Journal Book*, Portsmouth, NH: Heinemann.

Anderson, W. (1982) 'The use of journals in a human sexuality course', *Teaching of Psychology* **9**: 105–7.

Anon. (nd) 'Reflective journals of evidence', http://learning.unl.ac.uk/rtp/reflectivejournals.htm (accessed Aug 2005).

Armstong, L., Berry, M. and Lamshed, R. (nd) 'Blogs as electronic learning journals', http://www.usq.edu.au/electpub/ejist/docs/vol7_No1/CurrentPractice/Blogs.htm (accessed June 2005).

Ashbury, J., Fletcher, B. and Birtwhistle, R. (1993) 'Personal journal-writing in a communication course for first year medical students', *Medical Education* **27**: 196–204.

Aspinwall, K. (1986) 'Teacher biography: the in-service potential', *Cambridge Journal of Education* **16** (3): 210–15.

Ausubel, D. and Robinson, F. (1969) *School Learning*, London: Holt, Rhinehart and Winston.

Bales, R. (1957) *Interaction Process Analysis*, Reading, MA: Addison-Wesley.

Baltensperger, B. (1987) 'Journals in economic geography', in T. Fulwiler (ed.) *The Journal Book*, Portsmouth, NH: Heinemann.

Barnett, R. (1997) *Higher Education: a Critical Business*, Buckingham: Society for Research into Higher Education (SRHE)/Oxford University Press.

Baxter Magolda, M. (1992) *Knowing and Reasoning in College Students: Gender-related Patterns in Students' Intellectual Development*, San Francisco, CA: Jossey-Bass.

Baxter Magolda, M. (1994) 'Post college experiences and epistemology', *Review of Higher Education* **19**(1): 25–44.

Baxter Magolda, M. (1996) 'Epistemological development in graduate and professional education', *Review of Higher Education* **19**(3): 283–304.

Baxter Magolda, M. (1999) *Creating Contexts for Learning and Self Authorship*, San Francisco, CA: Jossey-Bass.

Baxter Magolda, M. (2001) *Making their Own Way*, Virginia, CA: Stylus.

Beard, C. and Wilson, J. (2002) *The Power of Experiential Learning*, London: RoutledgeFalmer.

Belenky, M., Clinchy, B., Goldberger, R. and Tarule, J. (1986) *Women's Ways of Knowing*, New York: Basic Books.

Bell, R. (1981) *Britain*, Glasgow: Collins.

Bennett, A. (2000) *Telling Tales*, London: Worldwide, BBC.

Berthoff, A. (1987) 'Dialectical notebooks and the audit of meaning', in T. Fulwiler (ed.) *The Journal Book*, Portsmouth, NH: Heinemann.

Betts, J. (2004) 'Theology, therapy or picket line? What's the "good" of reflective practice in management education?' *Reflective Practice* **5**(2): 239–51.

Biggs, J. and Collis, K. (1982) *Evaluating the Quality of Learning*, New York: Academic Press.

Bloom, B. (1956) *Taxonomy of Educational Objectives*, New York: Longmans-Green.

Boal, A. (1995) *The Rainbow of Desire*, London: Routledge.

Bolton, G. (1994) 'Stories at work: fictional-critical writing as a means of professional development', *British Journal of Educational Research* **20**(1): 55–68.

Bolton, G. (1999) *The Therapeutic Potential of Creative Writing – Writing Myself*, London: Jessica Kingsley.

Bolton, G. and Styles, M. (1995) 'There are stories and stories: an autobiographical workshop', in J. Swindells (ed.) *The Uses of Autobiography*, London: Taylor and Francis.

Boud, D. (2001) 'Using journal-writing to enhance reflective practice' in L. English and M. Gillen (eds) *Promoting Journal Writing in Adult Education: New Directions for Adult and Continuing Education*, no. 90, San Francisco, CA: Jossey-Bass.

Boud, D. and Miller, N. (eds) (1996) *Working with Experience*, London: Routledge.

Boud, D. and Walker, D. (1998) 'Promoting reflection in professional courses: the challenge of context', *Studies in Higher Education* **23**(2): 191–206.

Boud, D., Keogh, R. and Walker, D. (1985) *Reflection: Turning Experience into Learning*, London: Kogan Page.

Bowman, R. (1983) 'The personal student journal: mirror of the mind', *Contemporary Education* **55**: 25–7.

Bridges, W. (1980) *Transitions*, Reading, MA: Addison-Wesley.

Britton, J. (1972) 'Writing to learn and learning to write', in *The Humanity of English*, Urbana, IL: National Council of Teachers of English.

Brockbank, A. and McGill, I. (1998) *Facilitating Reflective Learning in Higher Education*, Buckingham: Society for Research into Higher Education (SRHE)/Oxford University Press.

Brodsky, D. and Meagher, E. (1987) 'Journals and political science', in T. Fulwiler (ed.) *The Journal Book*, Portsmouth, NH: Heinemann.

Brookfield, S. (1987) *Developing Critical Thinking*, Milton Keynes: Society for Research into Higher Education (SRHE)/Oxford University Press.

Brookfield, S. (1995) *Becoming a Critically Reflective Teacher*, San Francisco, CA: Jossey-Bass.

Brown, A., Ambruster, B. and Baker, L. (1986) 'The role of metacognition in reading and studying', in J. Orananu (ed.) *Reading Comprehension from Research to Practice*, Hillsdale, NJ: Lawrence Erlbaum.

Bruner, J. (1971) *The Relevance of Education*, New York: W. W. Norton.

Bruner, J. (1990) *Acts of Meaning*, Cambridge, MA: Harvard University Press.

Bunker, A. and Cronin, M. (1997) 'Improving students' academic writing with the use of the word processor', in R. Pospisil and L. Willcoxson (eds) *Learning Through Teaching*, pp. 50–7, proceedings of the 6th Annual Teaching Learning Forum, Murdoch University, February, Perth: Murdoch University. http://lsn.curtin.edu.au/tlf/tlf1997/bunker.html (accessed November 2005).

Burke, P. and Rainbow, B. (1998) 'Compile a portfolio', *Times Higher Educational Supplement*, 30 October.

Burnard, P. (1988) 'The journal as an assessment and evaluation tool in nurse education', *Nurse Education Today* **8**: 105–7.

Burnham, C. (1987) 'Reinvigorating a tradition: the personal development journal', in T. Fulwiler (ed.) *The Journal Book*, Portsmouth, NH: Heinemann.

Buzan, T. (1993) *The Mind Map Book*, London: BBC Books.

Calderhead, J. and James, C. (1992) 'Recording student teacher's learning experiences', *Journal of Further and Higher Education* **16**(1): 1–3.

Canning, C. (1991) 'What the teachers say about reflection', *Educational Leadership*, March.

Carlsmith, C. (1994) 'An "academical notebook"', http://www.trc.virginia.edu/ publications/teaching_concerns/spring 1994 (accessed November 2005).

Carr, W. and Kemmis, S. (1986) *Becoming Critical*, London: Falmer Press.

Cell, E. (1984) *Learning to Learn from Experience*, Albany, NY: State University of New York Press.

Chan, E. and Chuang, L. (2004) 'Teaching abstract concepts in contemporary nursing through spirituality', *Reflective Practice* **5**(1): 125.

Channel 4 (2005) *Big Brother* series, Summer, London: Channel 4.

Chi, M., Bassok, M., Lewis, M., Reimann, P. and Glaser, R. (1989) 'Self-explanations: how students study and use examples in learning to solve problems', *Cognitive Science* **13**: 145–82.

Chi, M., de Leeuw, N., Chiu, M. and LaVancher, C. (1994) 'Eliciting self-explanations improves learning', *Cognitive Science* **18**: 439–77.

Christensen, R. (1981) '"Dear diary", a learning tool for adults', *Lifelong Learning in the Adult Years* **October**: 158–62.

Clarke, B., James, C. and Kelly, J. (1996) 'Reflective practice, reviewing the issues and refocusing the debate', *International Journal of Nursing Studies* **33**(2): 171–80.

Claxton, G. (1999) *Wise Up: The Challenge of Lifelong Learning*, London: Bloomsbury.

Claxton, G. (2000) *The Intuitive Practitioner*, Milton Keynes: Open University Press.

Coltrinari, H. and Mitchell, C. (1999) 'Reflective journal-writing in the wired age', http://ww.oct.ca/english/ps/september_1999/journal.htm (accessed September 2005).

Connelly, F. and Clandinin, D. (1990) 'Stories of experience and narrative inquiry', *Educational Researcher* **19**(4): 2–14.

Cooper, J. (1991) 'Telling our own stories', in C. Whitehead and N. Noddings (eds) *Stories Lives Tell: Narrative and Dialogue in Education*, New York: Teacher's College Press.

Cottrell, S. (1999) *The Study Skills Handbook*, Basingstone: Macmillan.

Cottrell, S. (2003) *Skills for Success: Personal Development Planning Handbook*, London: Palgrave Macmillan.

Cowan, J. (1998a) Personal communication.

Cowan, J. (1998b) *On Becoming an Innovative University Teacher*, Buckingham: Society for Research into Higher Education (SRHE)/Oxford University Press.

Cowan, J. and Westwood, J. (2004) 'Collaborative and reflective professional development', unpublished paper (personal communication).

Creme, P. (1998) *New Forms of Student and Assessment in Social Anthropology: Research Through Practice at the University of Sussex*, National Network in Teaching and Learning Anthropology FDTL Project, 1997–98.

Crossley, M. (2002) 'Introducing narrative psychology', in C. Horrocks, K. Milnes, B. Roberts and D. Robinson (eds) *Narrative, Memory and Life Transitions*, Huddersfield: University of Huddersfield Press.

Csikszentmihalyi, M. (1990) *Flow: The Psychology of Optimal Experience*, New York: Harper and Row.

Damasio, A. (2000) *The Feeling of What Happens: Body, Emotion and the Making of Consciousness*, London: Virago.

Dart, B., Boulton-Lewis, G., Brownlee, J. and McCrindle, A. (1998) 'Change in knowledge of learning and teaching through journal-writing', *Research Papers in Education* 13(3): 291–318.

Davies, J. (1998) Paper given at *Improving Student Learning Conference*, Brighton.

Dawson, J. (2003) 'Reflectivy, creativity and the space for silence', *Reflective Practice* 4(1): 3–39.

Deshler, D. (1990) 'Conceptual mapping: drawing charts of the mind', in J. Mezirow (ed.) *Fostering Critical Reflection in Adulthood*, San Francisco, CA: Jossey-Bass.

Dewey, J. (1933) *How We Think*, Boston, MA: D. C. Heath and Co.

DiBiase, W. (1999) 'Have journal will travel: using travelling journals in science methods class', www.ed.psu/jounals/1999AETS/DiBiase.rft (accessed August 2005).

Didion, J. (1968) *Slouching Towards Bethlehem*, Harmondsworth: Penguin.

Dillon, D. (1983) 'Self-discovery through writing personal journals', *Language Arts* 60(3): 373–9.

Dimino, E. (1988) 'Clinical journals: a non-threatening strategy to foster ethical and intellectual development in nursing students', *Virginia Nurse* 56(1): 12–14.

Donaldson, M. (1992) *Human Minds: An Exploration*, Harmondsworth: Penguin.

Drake, S. and Elliot, A. (2005) 'Creating a new story to live by through collaborative reflection, concentric storying and using the old/new story framework', paper presented at the *Scenario-based Learning Conference*, Institute for Reflective Practice Gloucester.

Dunne, E. (2005) 'What does good teaching mean?' http://heacademy.ac.uk/profdev/LizDunnewhatdoesgoodteachingmean.rtf (accessed November 2005).

Eisner, E. (1991) 'Forms of understanding and the future of education', *Educational Researcher* 22: 5–11.

Elbow, P. (1973) *Writing without Teachers*, New York: Oxford University Press.

Elbow, P. (1981) *Writing with Power: Techniques for Mastering the Writing Process*, New York: Oxford University Press.

Elbow, P. and Clarke, J. (1987) 'Desert island discourse: the benefits of ignoring audience', in T. Fulwiler (ed.) *The Journal Book*, Portsmouth, NH: Heinemann.

Elkins, J. (1985) 'Rites of passage: law students "telling their lives"', *Journal of Legal Education* 35: 27–55.

Emig, J. (1977) 'Writing as a model of learning', *College Composition and Communication* 28: 122–8.

English, L. (2001) 'Ethical concerns relating to journal-writing', in L. English and M. Gillen, *Promoting Journal Writing in Adult Education: New Directions for Adult and Continuing Education*, no. 90, San Francisco, CA: Jossey-Bass.

English, L. and Gillen, M. (2001a) *Promoting Journal Writing in Adult Education: New Directions for Adult and Continuing Education*, no. 90, San Francisco, CA: Jossey-Bass.

English, L. and Gillen, M. (2001b) 'Journal-writing in practice; from vision to reality', in L. English and M. Gillen (eds) *Promoting Journal Writing in Adult Education: New Directions for Adult and Continuing Education*, no. 90, San Francisco, CA: Jossey-Bass.

Entwistle, N. (1996) 'Recent research on student learning and the learning environment', in J. Tait and P. Knight (eds) *The Management of Independent Learning*, London: SEDA/Kogan Page.

Eraut, M. (1994) *Developing Professional Knowledge and Competence*, London: Falmer Press.

Ertmer, P. and Newby, T. (1996) 'The expert learner: strategic, self-regulated and reflective', *Instructional Science* **24**: 1–24.

Evison, R. and Horobin, R. (1983) *How to Change Yourself and Your World: A Manual of Co-counselling*, Sheffield: Co-counselling Phoenix.

Fazey, D. (1993) 'Self-assessment as a genuine tool for enterprising students: the learning process', *Assessment and Evaluation in Higher Education* **18**(3): 335–50.

Fazey, J. and Marton, F. (2002) 'Understanding the space of experiential learning', *Active Learning in Higher Education* **3**(3): 234–50.

Fenwick, T. (2001) 'Responding to journals in a learning process', in L. English and M. Gillen (eds) *Promoting Journal Writing in Adult Education: New Directions for Adult and Continuing Education*, no. 90, San Francisco, CA: Jossey-Bass.

Ferry, N. and Ross-Gordon, J. (1998) 'An inquiry into Schön's epistemology of practice: exploring links between experiencing and workplace practice', *Adult Education Quarterly* **48**: 98–112.

Festinger, L. (1957) *A Theory of Cognitive Dissonance*, Stanford, CA: Stanford University Press.

Ficher, C. (1990) 'Student journal-writing in marketing courses', *Journal of Marketing Education* **Spring**: 46–51.

Field, J. (1952) *A Life of One's Own*, Harmondsworth: Penguin.

Finch, A. (1998) 'Designing and using a learner journal for false beginners: self-assessment and organization of learning', http://c.ust.hk/HASALD/newsletter/98newsletter (accessed November 2005).

Flavell, J. (1987) 'Speculations about the nature and development of metacognition', in F. Weincott and R. Kiuwe (eds), *Metacognition, Motivation and Understanding*, Hillsdale, NJ: Lawrence Erlbaum.

Flynn, E. (1986) 'Composing responses to literary texts', in A. Young and T. Fulwiler (eds) *Writing Across the Disciplines*, Upper Montclair, NJ: Boynton/Cook Publishers.

Fox, R. (1982) 'The personal log, enriching clinical practice', *Social Work Journal* **10**: 104–14.

Francis, D. (1995) 'Reflective journal: a window to preservice teachers' practical knowledge', *Teaching and Teacher Education* **11** (3): 229–41.

Fulwiler, T. (1986) 'Seeing with journals', *The English Record* **32**(3): 6–9.

Fulwiler, T. (1987) *The Journal Book*, Portsmouth, NH: Heinemann.

Furedi, F. (2005) 'I refuse to hand it to students on a plate', *Times Higher Educational Supplement*, 25 March.

Gatlin, L. (1987) 'Losing control and liking it: journals in Victorian literature', in T. Fulwiler (ed.) *The Journal Book*, Portsmouth, NH: Heinemann.

Gelter, H. (2003) 'Why is reflective thinking uncommon?', *Reflective Practice* 4(3): 337–44.

Gersie, A. and King, N. (1990) *Storymaking in Education and Therapy*, London: Jessica Kingsley.

Ghaye, A. and Lillyman, S. (1997) *Learning Journals and Critical Incidents*, Dinton: Quay Books.

Gibbs, G. (1988) *Learning by Doing: A Guide to Teaching and Learning Methods*, Birmingham: Standing Conference for Educational Development (SCED).

Gillis, A. (2001) 'Journal-writing in health education', in L. English and M. Gillen, *Promoting Journal Writing in Adult Education: New Directions for Adult and Continuing Education*, no. 90, San Francisco, CA: Jossey-Bass.

Glaze, J. (2002) 'PhD Study and the use of a reflective diary: a dialogue with self', *Reflective Practice* 3(2): 153–66.

Goleman, D. (1995) *Emotional Intelligence*, New York: Bantam Books.

Goleman, D. (1998) *Working with Emotional Intelligence*, London: Bloomsbury.

Gough, N. (1993) 'Environmental education, narrative complexity and postmodern science/fiction', *International Journal of Science Education* 15(5): 607–25.

Grainger, R. (1997) *Traditional Storytelling in the Primary Classroom*, Leamington Spa: Scholastic Books.

Greenhalgh, T. (1998) 'The conker tree', in T. Greenhalgh and B. Hurwitz (eds) *Narrative Based Medicine*, London: British Medical Journal.

Greenhalgh, T. and Collard, A. (2003) *Narrative-based Healthcare: Sharing Stories*, London: British Medical Journal.

Greenhalgh, T. and Hurwitz, B. (1998) 'Why study narrative?', in T. Greenhalgh and B. Hurwitz (eds) *Narrative Based Medicine*, London: British Medical Journal.

Griffiths, M. and Tann, S. (1992) 'Using reflective practice to link personal and public theories', *Journal of Education for Teaching* 18(11): 69–83.

Grumbacher, J. (1987) 'How writing helps physics students become better problem solvers', in T. Fulwiler (ed.) *The Journal Book*, Portsmouth, NH: Heinemann.

Grumet, M. (1987) 'The polities of personal knowledge', *Curriculum Inquiry* 17(13): 9–35.

Grumet, M. (1989) 'Generations: reconceptualist curriculum theory and teacher education', *Journal of Teacher Education* **January-February**:13–17.

Grumet, M. (1990) 'Retrospective: autobiography and the analysis of educational experience', *Cambridge Journal of Education* 20(3): 321–5.

Gundmundsdottir, S. (1995) 'The narrative nature of pedagogical content knowledge', in H. McEwan and H. Egan (eds) *Narrative in Teaching, Learning and Research*, New York: Teacher's College Press.

Habermas, J. (1971) *Knowledge and Human Interests*, London: Heinemann.

Hadwin, A. and Winne, P. (1996) 'Study strategies have meagre support: a review with recommendations for implementation', *Journal of Higher Education* 67(6): 1–17.

Hahnemann, B. (1986) 'Journal-writing: a way to promoting critical thinking in nursing students', *Journal of Nursing Education* 25(5): 213–15.

Hallberg, F. (1987) 'Journal-writing as person-making', in T. Fulwiler (ed.) *The Journal Book*, Portsmouth, NH: Heinemann.

Handley, P. (1998) Personal communication.

Hartley, J. (1998) *Learning and Studying*, London: Routledge.

Harvey, L. and Knight, P. (1996) *Transforming Higher Education*, Buckingham: Society for Research into Higher Education (SRHE)/Oxford University Press.

Hatton, N. and Smith, D. (1995) 'Reflection in teacher education: towards definition and implementation', *Teaching and Teacher Education* 11(1): 33–49.

HEA, HEBS, HPW, HPANI (1995) *Handbook on the Development of Foundation Courses in Health Promotion*, Cardiff: Health Promotion Wales.

Heath, H. (1998) 'Keeping a reflective practice diary: a practical guide', *Nurse Education Today* 18(18): 592–98.

Hiemstra, R. (2001) 'Uses and benefits of journal-writing', in L. English and M. Gillen (eds) *Promoting Journal Writing in Adult Education: New Directions for Adult and Continuing Education*, no. 90, San Francisco, CA: Jossey-Bass.

Hesse, H. (1975) *Autobiographical Writing*, London: Picador.

Hettich, P. (1976) 'The journal, an autobiographical approach to learning', *Teaching of Psychology* 3(2): 60–1.

Hettich, P. (1980) 'The evaluator's journal', *CEDR Quarterly* 13(2): 19–22.

Hettich, P. (1988) 'Journal-writing: an autobiographical approach to learning', *High School Psychology Teacher* 19(3): 416–17.

Hettich, P. (1990) 'Journal-writing: old fare or nouvelle cuisine?', *Teaching of Psychology* 17(1): 36–9.

Hickman, K. (1987) 'There's a place for the log in the office', in T. Fulwiler (ed.) *The Journal Book*, Portsmouth, NH: Heinemann.

Hinett, K. (2003) *Improving Learning Through Reflection, Parts 1, 2*, reprinted from the Institute for Learning and Teaching in Higher Education (ILTHE) members' website (http://www.ilt.ac.uk (not now available).

Holden, E. (1977) *The Country Diary of an Edwardian Lady*, London: Michael Joseph, Webb and Bower.

Holly, M. (1989) 'Reflective writing and the spirit of inquiry', *Cambridge Journal of Education* 19(1): 71–80.

Holly, M. (1991) *Keeping a Personal-Professional Journal*, Geelong, Victoria, Australia: Deakin University Press.

Holly, M. and McLoughlin, C. (1989) *Perspectives on Teacher Professional Development*, London: Falmer Press.

Hoover, L. (1994) 'Reflective writing as a window on pre-service teachers' thought processes', *Teaching and Teacher Education* 10: 83–93.

Houghton, P. (1998) *Learning from Work*, Module workbook CD2006, Preston, Lancs: University of Central Lancashire.

Hunt, C. (1998) 'Writing with the voice of the child', in C. Hunt and F. Sampson (eds) *The Self on the Page*, London: Jessica Kingsley.

Hunt, C. (2000) *Therapeutic Dimensions of Autobiography*, London: Jessica Kingsley.

Hunt, C. and Sampson, F. (1998) *The Self on the Page*, London: Jessica Kingsley.

Hunt, D. (1987) *Beginning with Ourselves*, Cambridge, MA: Brookline Books.

Hutton, P. (2004) *I Would Not Be Forgotten: The Life and Works of Robert Stephen Hawker*, Padstow, Cornwall: Tabb House.

Institute for Reflective Practice (2005) www.reflectivepractices.co.uk/cms/index.php.

Jacobson, A. (nd) 'Essential learning skills across the curriculum', Oregon State Department of Education, http://www.sdcoe.K12.ca.us/score/actbnank/tjourlact.htm (accessed November 2005).

Jakins, H. (1970) *Fundamentals of Co-Counselling*, revised edn, Washington: Rational Island.

James, C. (1993) 'Developing reflective practice skills: the potential', paper presented to *The Power of the Portfolio Conference*, London.

James, C. and Denley, P. (1993) 'Using records of experience in an undergraduate certificate in education course', *Evaluation and Research in Education* **6**: 23–37.

Jasper, M. (1998) 'Assessing and improving student outcomes through reflective writing', in C. Rust (ed.) *Improving Student Learning*, Oxford: Oxford Centre for Staff and Learning Development (OCSLD), Oxford Brookes University, pp. 1–15.

Jaye, J. (2001) 'Learning from holiday and emotional events', unpublished (some personal writing; personal communication).

Jaye, J. (2005) personal communication.

Jensen, E. (1979) 'Student journals in the social problems course: applying sociological concepts', paper presented at the annual meeting of the Pacific Sociological Association.

Jensen, V. (1987) 'Writing in college physics', in T. Fulwiler (ed.) *The Journal Book*, Portsmouth, NH: Heinemann.

Johns, C. (1994) 'Nuances of recollection', *Journal of Clinical Nursing* **3**: 71–5.

Joyce, M. (nd) 'Double entry journals and learning logs', http://www.mslibraries.org/infolit/ samplers/spring/doub.html (accessed November 2005).

Jung, C. (1961) *Memories, Dreams and Reflections*, New York: Random House.

Kaiser, R. (1981) 'The way of the journal', *Psychology Today* **March**: 64–76.

Kallaith, T. and Coghlan, D. (2003) 'Developing reflective skills through journal-writing in an OD course', *Organisational Development Journal* **10**(4): 61–9.

Kelly, G. (1955) *The Psychology of Personal Construct Theory*, New York: W. W. Norton.

Kember, D., Jones, A., Loke, A., McKay, J., Sinclair, K., Harrison, T., Webb, C., Wong, F. and Yeung, F. (1999) 'Determining the level of reflective thinking from student's written journals using a coding scheme based on Mezirow', *International Journal of Lifelong Learning* **18**(1): 18–30.

Kember, D., Leung, D., with Jones, A., Loke, A., McKay, J., Harrison, T., Webb, C., Wong, F. and Yeung, F. (2000) 'Development of a questionnaire to measure the level of reflective thinking', *Assessment and Evaluation in Higher Education* **25**(4): 370–80.

Kent, O. (1987) 'Student journals and the goals of philosophy', in T. Fulwiler (ed.) *The Journal Book*, Portsmouth, NH: Heinemann.

Kenyon, G., Clarke, P. and De Vries, B. (2001) *Narrative Gerontology*, New York: Springer Publishing.

Kim, H. (1999) 'Critical reflective inquiry for knowledge development in nursing practice', *Journal of Advanced Nursing* **29**(5): 1205–12.

King, P. and Kitchener, K. (1994) *Developing Reflective Judgement*, San Francisco, CA: Jossey-Bass.

Kneale, P. (1997) 'The rise of the "strategic student": how can we cope?', in M. Armstrong, G. Thompson and S. Brown (eds) *Facing up to Radical Changes in Universities and Colleges*, London: Staff and Educational Development Association (SEDA)/Kogan Page.

Knowles, J. (1993) 'Life history accounts as mirrors: a practical avenue for the conceptualization of reflection in teacher education', in J. Calderhead and P. Gates (eds) *Conceptualizing Development in Teacher Education*, London: Falmer Press.

Kolb, D. (1984) *Experiential Learning as the Science of Learning and Development*, Englewood Cliffs, NJ: Prentice Hall.

Korthagan, F. (1988) 'The influence of learning orientation on the development of reflective teaching', in J. Calderhead (ed.) *Teachers' Professional Learning*, London: Falmer Press.

Lamarque, P. (1990) 'Narrative and invention: the limits of fictionality', in C. Nash (ed.) *Narrative in Culture*, London: Routledge.

Landeen, J., Byrne, C. and Brown, B. (1992) 'Journal-keeping as an educational strategy in learning psychiatric nursing', *Journal of Advanced Nursing* **17**: 347–55.

Lave, J. and Wenger, E. (1991) *Situated Learning: Legitimate Peripheral Participation*, Cambridge: Cambridge University Press.

Lea, M. and Stierer, B. (2000) *Student Writing in Higher Education*, Buckingham: Society for Research into Higher Education (SRHE)/Oxford University Press.

Lea, M. and Street, B. (2000) 'Student writing and staff feedback in higher education: an academic literacies approach', in M. Lea and B. Stierer (eds) *Student Writing in Higher Education*, Buckingham: Society for Research into Higher Education (SRHE)/Oxford University Press.

Ledwith, M. (2005) 'Personal narratives/political lives: a personal reflection as a tool for reflective change', *Reflective Practice* **6**(2): 255–62.

Lindberg, A. (1955) *Gift from the Sea*, New York: Pantheon Books.

Lindberg, G. (1987) 'The journal conference: from dialectic to dialogue', in T. Fulwiler (ed.) *The Journal Book*, Portsmouth, NH: Heinemann.

Linden, J. (1999) 'The contribution of narrative to the process of supervising PhD students', *Studies in Higher Education* **24**(3): 351–64.

Lipman, D. (2003) 'Can the "story mind" be trained? E-tips on storytelling', bounce.sc @storytellingcoach.com (accessed 2003).

Longenecker, R. (2002) 'The jotter wallet: invoking reflective practice in a family practice residency programme', *Reflective Practice* **3**(2): 219–24.

Lowenstein, S. (1987) 'A brief history of journal keeping', in T. Fulwiler (ed.) *The Journal Book*, Portsmouth, NH: Heinemann.

Lucas, B. (2001) *Power up Your Mind*, London: Nicholas Brealey.

Lukinsky, J. (1990) 'Reflective withdrawal through journal-writing', in J. Mezirow (ed.) *Fostering Critical Reflection in Adulthood*, San Francisco, CA: Jossey-Bass.

Lyons, J. (1999) 'Reflective education for professional practice: discovering knowledge from experience', *Nurse Education Today* **19**: 29–34.

McAlpine, L. and Weston, C. (2002) 'Reflection, improving teaching and students learning', in N. Hativa and P. Goodyear (eds) *Teacher Thinking Beliefs and Knowledge in Higher Education*, Dordrecht: Kluwer Academic Publishers, pp: 59–77.

McCanch, N. (1985) *A Lighthouse Notebook*, London: Michael Joseph.

McCrindle, A. and Christensen, C. (1995) 'The impact of learning journals on metacognitive processes and learning performance', *Learning and Instruction* **5**(3): 167–85.

McDrury, J. and Alterio, M. (2003) *Learning through Storytelling*, London: Routledge-Falmer.

Mackintosh, C. (1998) 'Reflection: a flawed strategy for the nursing profession', *Nurse Education Today* **18**: 553–7.

McManus, J. (1986) 'Live case study, journal record in adolescent psychology', *Teaching of Psychology* **13**: 70–4.

Macrorie, K. (1970) *Uptake*, Rochelle Park, NJ: Hayden Book Company.

Mallon, T. (1984) *A Book of One's Own: People and Their Diaries*, New York: Ticknor and Fields.

Mansfield, S. and Bidwell, L. (2005) 'The use of creative writing techniques in developing students' use of reflexive journals', session at Dundee University Staff Development day, 27 June.

Martin, J. (1998) Personal communication.

Marton, F. and Booth, S. (1997) *Learning and Awareness*, Hillsdale, NJ: Lawrence Erlbaum.

Marton, F., Hounsell, D. and Entwistle, N. (1997) *The Experience of Learning*, Edinburgh: Academic Press.

Mayher, J., Lester, N. and Pradl, M. (1983) *Learning to Write, Writing to Learn*, Upper Montclair, NJ: Boynton/Cook.

Meese, G. (1987) 'Focused leaning in chemistry research: Suzanne's journal', in T. Fulwiler (ed.) *The Journal Book*, Portsmouth, NH: Heinemann.

Mezirow, J. (1998) 'On critical reflection', *Adult Education Quarterly* **48**(3): 185–99.

Miller, J. (1983) 'A search for congruence: influence of past and present in future teachers' concepts about teaching writing', *English Education* **15 February**: 5–16.

Miller, J. (1987) 'Teacher's emerging texts: the empowering potential of writing in service', in J. Smyth (ed.) *Educating Teachers*, London: Falmer Press.

Miller, S. (1979) 'Keeping a psychological journal', *The Gifted Child Quarterly* **23**: 168–75.

Milner, M. (1957) *On Not Being Able to Paint*, London: Heinemann.

Milner, M. (1987) *Eternity's Sunrise: A Way of Keeping a Diary*, London: Virago.

Moon, J. (1996b) 'Generic level descriptors and their place in the standards debate', *Focus* **Autumn**: 64–9. London:

Moon, J. (1996a) 'What can you do in a day? Advice on developing short training courses on promoting health', *Journal of the Institute of Health Promotion* **34**(1): 20–3.

Moon, J. (1999a) *Reflection in Learning and Professional Development*, London: RoutledgeFalmer.

Moon, J. (1999b) *Learning Journals: A Handbook for Academics, Students and Professional Development*, London: RoutledgeFalmer (first edition).

Moon, J. (1999c) 'Describing higher education: some conflicts and conclusions', in H. Smith, M. Armstrong and S. Brown (eds) *Benchmarking and Threshold Standards in Higher Education*, London: Staff and Educational Development Association (SEDA)/ Kogan Page.

Moon, J. (2002) *A Handbook of Module and Programme Development*, London: RoutledgeFalmer.

Moon, J. (2004a) *A Handbook of Reflective and Experiential Learning*, London: RoutledgeFalmer.

Moon, J. (2004b) 'Information from interviews with students: a programme that takes lay people to the Ministry (SW Ministry programme)', unpublished paper.

Moon, J. (2004c) 'Using reflective learning to improve the impact of short courses and workshops', *Journal of Continuing Education in the Health Professions* **24**(1): 4–11.

Moon, J. (2005a) 'They seek it here. A new perspective on the elusive activity of critical thinking: a theoretical and practical approach', Higher Education Academy Subject Centre for Education website, www.ESCalate.ac.uk. Also available as a paper publication (43 pages) from ESCalate, Univerisity of Bristol.

Moon, J. (2005b) 'Coming from behind: an investigation of learning issues in the process of widening participation in higher education', Final Report (March), Higher Education Academy Subject Centre for Education, www.ESCalate.ac.uk/index.cfm?action=grants. completed (accessed January 2006).

Moon, J. (2005c) 'Putting writing at the centre', *Bulletin*, Spring 2005, Higher Education Academy Subject Centre for Education (ESCalate), www.ESCalate.ac.uk

Moon, J. (2005d) 'First person', unpublished short story.

Moon, J. and England, P. (1994) 'The development of a highly structured workshop in health promotion', *Journal of the Institute of Health Education* 32(2): 41–4.

Morgan, N. and Saxon, S. (1991) *Teaching Questioning and Learning*, London: Routledge.

Morrison, K. (1990) *Learning Logs*, Durham: Department of Education, University of Durham.

Morrison, K. (1996) 'Developing reflective practice in higher degree students through a learning journal', *Studies in Higher Education* 21(3): 317–32.

Mortiboys, A. (2002) 'The emotionally intelligent lecturer', *Staff and Educational Development Association (SEDA) Special Paper* 12, Birmingham: SEDA.

Mortimer, J. (1998) 'Motivating student learning through facilitating independence: self and peer assessment of reflective practice - an action research project', in S. Brown, S. Armstrong and G. Thompson (eds) *Motivating Students*, London: Staff and Educational Development Association (SEDA)/Kogan Page.

Mülhaus, S. and Löschmann, M. (1997) 'Improving independent learning with aural German programmes', in R. Hudson, S. Maslin-Prothero and L. Oates (eds) *Flexible Learning in Action*, London: SEDA/Kogan Page.

National Institute for Careers Education and Counselling (NICEC) (1998) 'Developing career management skills in higher education', *Briefing*, NICEC, Sheraton House, Castle Park, Cambridge.

National Committee of Inquiry into Higher Education (NCIHE) (1997) *Report (The Dearing Report)*, London: NCIHE.

Neary, M. (1998) Personal communication.

Neelands, J. (1992) *Learning though Imagined Experience: The Role of Drama in the National Curriculum*, London: Hodder and Stoughton.

Neopolitan, J. (2004) 'Doing professional development school work: a tale of heroes, allies and dragons at the door', *Reflective Practice* 5(1).

Nisbett, R.and DeCamp Wilson, T. (1977) 'Telling more than we can know: verbal reports on mental processes', *Psychological Review* 84(3): 231–57.

Noddings, N. (1996) 'Stories and affect in teacher education', *Cambridge Journal of Education* 26(3): 435–47.

November, P. (1993) 'Journals for the journey into deep learning', *Research and Development in Higher Eeducation* 16: 299–303.

Nymark, S. (2000) *Organisational Storytelling*, Oslo: Foglaget Ankerhus.

Oberg, A. and Underwood, S. (1992) 'Facilitative self development: reflections on experience', in A. Hargreaves and M. Fulton (eds) *Understanding Teacher Development*, New York: Teacher's College Press.

Oliver, R. (1998) Personal communication.

Orem, R. (2001) 'Journal-writing in adult ESL: improving practice through reflective writing', in L. English and M. Gillen (eds) *Promoting Journal Writing in Adult Education: New Directions for Adult and Continuing Education*, no. 90, San Francisco, CA: Jossey-Bass.

Paris, S. and Winograd, P. (1990) 'How metacognition can promote academic learning and instruction', in B. Jones and L. Idol (eds) *Dimensions of Thinking and Cognitive Instruction*, Hillsdale, NJ: Lawrence Erlbaum.

Parker, R. and Goodkin, V. (1987) *The Consequences of Writing: Enhancing Learning in the Disciplines*, Upper Montclair, NJ:Boynton/Cook.

Parnell, J. (1998) Personal communication.

Paul, R. (1990) 'Critical and reflective thinking: a philosophical perspective', in B. Jones and L. Idol (eds) *Dimensions of Thinking and Cognitive Instruction*, Hillsdale, NJ: Lawrence Erlbaum Associates.

Paulson, T., Paulson, P. and Meyer, C. (1991) 'What makes a portfolio a portfolio?', *Educational Leadership* **February**: 60–5.

Perry, W. (1970) *Forms of Intellectual and Academic Developments in College Years*, New York: Holt, Rhinehart and Winston.

Peterson, E. and Jones, A. (2001) 'Women, journal-writing and the reflective process', in L. English and M. Gillen (eds) *Promoting Journal Writing in Adult Education: New Directions for Adult and Continuing Education*, no. 90, San Francisco, CA: Jossey-Bass.

Piaget, J. (1971) *Biology and Knowledge*, Edinburgh: Edinburgh University Press.

Pinar, W. (1975) 'Currere: towards reconceptualization', in W. Pinar (ed.) *Curriculum Theorizing*, Berkeley, CA: McCutcham.

Prawat, R. (1989) 'Promoting access to knowledge, strategy and disposition in students: a research synthesis', *Review of Educational Research* **50**(1): 1–41.

Prawat, R. (1991) 'Conversations with self and settings', *American Educational Research Journal* **28**(4): 737–57.

Progoff, I. (1975) *At a Journal Workshop*, New York: Dialogue House Library.

Progoff, I. (1980) *The Practice of Process Meditation* New York: Dialogue House Library.

Quality Assurance Agency (QAA) (2000) 'Policy statements for progress files for higher education', http://www.qaa.ac.uk/academicinfrastructure/progressfiles/guidelines/policy statement/default/asp (accessed November 2005).

Rainer, T. (1978) *The New Diary. How to Use a Journal for Self Guidance and Extended Creativity*, N. Ryde, NSW, Australia: Angus and Robertson.

Rainwater, J. (1983) *You're in Charge*, Wellingborough: Turnstone Press.

Rarieya, J. (2005) 'Promoting and investigating students' uptake of reflective practice', *Relfective Practice* **6**(2): 285–94.

Redwine, M. (1989) 'The autobiography as a motivating factor for students', in S. Warner Weil and I. McGill (eds) *Making Sense of Experiential Learning*, Buckingham: Society for Research into Higher Education (SRHE)/Oxford University Press.

Reid, A. and Leigh, E. (1998) 'Three dimensional images in self assessment of learning', paper presented at *Improving Student Learning Conference*, Brighton University, September.

Richardson, L. (1994) 'Writing: a method of inquiry', in N. Denzil and Y. Lincoln (eds) *Handbook of Qualitative Research*, London: Sage.

Richardson, V. (1997) 'Constructiveness teaching and teacher education: theory and practice', in V. Richardson (ed.) *Constructivist Teacher Education*, London: Falmer Press.

Ricoeur, P. (1984) *Time and Narrative*, Chicago, IL: University of Chicago Press.

Roderick, J. (1986) 'Dialogue journal-writing: context for reflecting on self as teacher and researcher', *Journal Curriculum and Supervision* **1**(4): 305–15.

Roderick, J. and Berman, L. (1984) 'Dialoguing and dialogue journals', *Language Arts* **61**(7): 686–92.

Rogers, C. (1969) *Freedom to Learn*, Columbus, OH: Charles E. Merrill.

Ross, D. (1989) 'First steps in developing a reflective approach', *Journal of Teacher Education* **40**(2): 22–30.

Rothwell, A. and Ghelipter, S. (2003) 'The developing manager: reflective learning in undergraduate management education', *Reflective Practice* **4**(2): 240–54.

Rovegno, I. (1992) 'Learning to reflect on teaching: a case study of one preservice physical education teacher', *The Elementary School Journal* **92**(4): 491–510.

Rowling, J. (2000) *Harry Potter and the Goblet of Fire*, London: Bloomsbury.

Sagor, R. (1991) 'What project LEARN reveals about corroborative action research', *Educational Leadership* **March**: 6–9.

Salisbury, J. (1994) 'Becoming qualified: an ethnography of a post-experience teacher-training course', PhD thesis, University College of Wales, Cardiff.

Samuals, M. and Betts, J. (2005) 'Crossing the threshold from description to deconstruction: using self assessment to deepen reflection on lived scenarios', paper presented at *Institute of Reflective Practice Conference*, June, 'Scenario-Based Learning', Gloucester.

Sanford, B. (1988) 'Writing reflectively', *Language Arts* **65**(7): 652–57.

Schneider, M. and Killick, J. (1998) *Writing for Self Discovery*, Shaftsbury: Element Books.

Schön, D. (1983) *The Reflective Practitioner*, San Francisco, CA: Jossey-Bass.

Schön, D. (1987) *Educating the Reflective Practitioner*, San Francisco, CA: Jossey-Bass.

Selfe, C. and Arbabi, F. (1986) 'Writing to learn: engineering students journals', in A. Young and T. Fulwiler (eds) *Writing Across the Disciplines*, Upper Montclair, NJ: Boynton/Cook.

Selfe, C., Petersen, B. and Nahrgang, C. (1986) 'Journal-writing in mathematics', in A. Young and T. Fulwiler (eds) *Writing Across the Disciplines*, Upper Montclair, NJ: Boynton/Cook.

Shepherd, M. (2004) 'Reflections on developing a reflective journal as a management advisor', *Reflective Practice* **5**(2): 199–204.

Shohet, R. (1985) *Dream Sharing*, Wellingborough: Turnstone Press.

Smyth, J. (1987) *Changing the Nature of Pedagogical Knowledge*, Lewes: Falmer Press.

Smyth, J. (1989) 'Developing and sustaining critical reflection in teacher education', *Journal Teacher Education* **40**(2): 2–9.

Snowden, D. (2003) 'Narrative patterns: the perils and possibilities of using story in organizations', in E. Lesser, and K. Prusak (eds) *Creating Value with Knowledge*, Oxford: Oxford University Press.

Sparkes, A. (2002) *Telling Tales in Sport and Activity*, Leeds: Human Kinetics.

Sparkes-Langer, G. and Colton, A. (1991) 'Synthesis of research on teachers' reflective thinking', *Educational Leadership* **March**: 37–44.

Sparkes-Langer, G., Simmons, J., Pasch, M., Colton, A. and Starko, A. (1990) 'Reflective peda-gogical thinking: how can we promote and measure it?', *Journal of Teacher Education* **41**: 23–32.

Staton, J. (1988) 'Contributions of the dialogue journal research to communicating, thinking and learning', in J. Staton, R. Shuy, S. Peyton and L. Reed (eds) *Dialogue Journal Communication*, Norwood, NJ: Ablex.

Staton, J., Shuy, R., Peyton, S. and Reed, L. (eds) (1988) *Dialogue Journal Communication*, Norwood, NJ: Ablex.

Steffens, H. (1987) 'Journals in the teaching of history', in T. Fulwiler (ed.) *The Journal Book*, Portsmouth, NH: Heinemann.

Stephani, L. (1997) 'Reflective teaching in higher education', *Universites' and Colleges' Staff Development Agency (UCoSDA) Briefing Paper* **42**, Sheffield: UCoSDA.

Stephani, L., Clarke, J. and Littlejohn, A. (2000) 'Developing a student-centred approach to reflective leaning', *Innovations in Education and Training International* **27**(2): 63–169.

Stephani, L. (1999) 'Reflections on self control', *Times Higher Educational Supplement*, 16 April.

Stockhausen, L. and Kawashima, A. (2002) 'The introduction of reflective practice to Japanese nurses', *Reflective Practice* **3**(1): 117–28.

Storr, A. (1988) *Solitude*, London: Flamingo.

Sumsion, J. and Fleet, A. (1996) 'Reflection: can we assess it? Should we assess it?', *Assessment and Evaluation in Higher Education* **21**(2): 121–30.

Surbeck, E., Han, . and Moyer, J. (1991) 'Assessing reflective responses in journals', *Educational Leadership* **March**: 25–7.

Talbot, M. (2002) 'Reflective practice: new insights or more of the same? Thoughts on an autobiographicl critical incident analysis', *Reflective Practice* **3**(2): 225–29.

Tama, C. and Peterson, K. (1991) 'Achieving reflectivity through literature', *Educational Leadership* **March**: 22–4.

Taylor, C. and White, S. (2000) *Practising Reflectivity in Health and Welfare*, Milton Keynes: Open University Press.

Taylor, E. (1997) 'Building upon the theoretical debate: a critical review of the empirical studies of Mezirow's transformative learning debate', *Adult Education Quarterly* **48**(1): 34–59.

Terry, W. (1984) 'A "forgetting" journal for memory courses', *Teaching of Psychology* **11**: 111–12.

Thorpe, K. (2004) 'Learning journals: from concept to practice', *Reflective Practice* **5**(3): 339–45.

Tomlinson, P. (1999) 'Continuous reflection and implicit learning: towards a balance in teacher preparation', *Oxford Review of Education* **25**(4): 533–44.

Trelfa, J. (2005) 'Faith in reflective practice', *Reflective Practice* **6**(2): 205–12.

Tripp, D. (1987) 'Teacher's journals and collaborative research', in J. Smyth (ed.) *Changing the Nature of Pedagogical Knowledge*, Lewes: Falmer Press.

Tsang, W. (2003) 'Journaling from internship to practice teaching', *Reflective Practice* **4**(2): 221–40.

Van Manen, M. (1977) 'Linking ways of knowing and ways of being', *Curriculum Inquiry* **6**: 205–8.

Van Rossum, E. and Schenk, S. (1984) 'The relationship between learning conception, study strategy and learning outcome', *British Journal of Educational Psychology* **54**: 73–83.

Voss, M. (1988) 'The light at the end of the journal: a teacher learns about learning', *Language Arts* **65**(7): 669–74.

Vygotsky, L. (1978) *Mind in Society: the Development of Higher Psychological Processes*, Cambridge, MA: Harvard University Press.

Wagenaar, T. (1984) 'Using student journals in sociology courses', *Teaching Sociology* **11**: 419–37.

Walker, D. (1985) 'Writing and reflection', in D. Boud, R. Keogh and D. Walker (eds) *Reflection: Turning Experience into Learning*, London: Kogan Page.

Wedman, J. and Martin, M. (1986) 'Exploring the development of reflective thinking through journal-writing', *Reading Improvement* **23**(1): 68–71.

Weil, S. (1996) 'From the other side of science: new possibilities for dialogue in academic writing', *Changes* **3**: 223–31.

Weinstein, C. (1987) 'Fostering learning autonomy through the use of learning strategies', *Journal Reading* **7**: 590–95.

Wellington, B. (1991) 'The promise of reflective practice', *Educational Leadership* **March**: 4–5.

West, H. and Pines, A.(1985) *Cognitive Structure and Conceptual Change*, New York: Academic Press.

Wetherell, J. and Mullins, G. (nd) 'Drilling for gold', http://www.adelaide.edu.au/clpd/material/leap/case_studies/wetherell.html (accessed November 2005).

Wetherell, J. and Mullins, G. (1996) 'The use of student journals in problem-based learning', *Medical Education* **30**: 105–11.

Whelan, K., Huber, J., Rose, C., Davies, A. and Clandinin, D. (2001) 'Telling and retelling our stories on the professional development landscape', *Teachers and Teaching: Theory and Practice* **7**(2): 143–56.

Wildman, T. and Niles, J. (1987) 'Reflective teachers, tensions between abstractions and realities', *Journal of Teacher Education* **3**: 25–31.

Wilkes, A. (1997) *Knowledge in Minds: Individual and Collective Processes in Cognition*, London: Psychology Press.

Wilkinson, J. and Robb, A. (nd) 'SCL case study interviews assessment methods: reflective journal', http://www.gla.ac.uk/services/tls/ProjectReports/Case/Reflective/ (accessed June 2005).

Winitzky, N. and Kauchak, D. (1997) 'Constructivism in teacher education: applying cognitive theory to teacher learning', in V. Richardson (ed.) *Constructivist Teacher Education*, London: Falmer Press.

Winter, R., Buck, A. and Sobiechowska, P. (1999) *Professional Experience and the Investigative Imagination*, London: Routledge.

Wolf Moondance (1994) *Rainbow Medicine*, New York: Sterling.

Wolf, J. (1980) 'Experiential learning in professional education: concepts and tools', *New Directions for Experiential Learning* **8**: 1–26.

Wolf, M. (1989) 'Journal-writing: a means to an end in educating students to work with older adults', *Gerontology and Geriatrics Education* **10**: 53–62.

Wolf, V. (1978*) A Writer's Diary*, London: Triad/Granada.

Woods, P. (1987) 'Life histories and teacher knowledge', in J. Smyth (ed.) *Educating Teachers: Changing the Nature of Pedagogical Knowledge*, Lewes: Falmer Press.

Woolf, V. (1929) *A Room of One's Own*, Harmondsworth: Penguin.

Yinger, R. (1985) 'Journal-writing as a learning tool', *The Volta Review* **87**(5): 21–33.

Yinger, R. and Clark, M. (1981) 'Reflective journal-writing: theory and practice', Occasional Paper no. 50, East Lansing, Michigan State University Institute for Research on Teaching.

Young, A. and Fulwiler, T. (1986) *Writing Across the Disciplines*, Upper Montclair, NJ: Boynton/Cook.

Index